THE EFFECTS

Founded by C. K. Ogden

The International Library of Psychology

COGNITIVE PSYCHOLOGY
In 21 Volumes

THE EFFECTS OF MUSIC

A Series of Essays

Edited by MAX SCHOEN

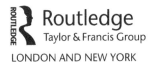

Routledge
Taylor & Francis Group

LONDON AND NEW YORK

First published in 1927 by
Routledge, Trench, Trubner & Co., Ltd.
2 Park Square, Milton Park, Abingdon, Oxfordshire OX14 4RN
711 Third Avenue, New York, NY 10017

First issued in paperback 2014

Routledge is an imprint of the Taylor and Francis Group, an informa business

British Library Cataloguing in Publication Data
A CIP catalogue record for this book
is available from the British Library

The Effects of Music
ISBN 0415-20973-0
Cognitive Psychology: 21 Volumes
ISBN 0415-21126-3
The International Library of Psychology: 204 Volumes
ISBN 0415-19132-7

ISBN 13: 978-1-138-87506-7 (pbk)
ISBN 13: 978-0-415-20973-1 (hbk)

ACKNOWLEDGMENT

The Editor wishes to acknowledge his indebtedness to the investigators whose studies appear in this volume for their generous co-operation, and to the editors of the *British Journal of Psychology*, the *Journal of Applied Psychology*, the *Journal of Experimental Psychology*, for permission to reprint the studies of Dr. Myers, Drs. Gilliland and Moore, and Dr. Hyde, respectively.

M. S.

PITTSBURGH,
January, 1927.

CONTENTS

CONTENTS

SECTION III

THE MOOD EFFECTS OF MUSIC

SECTION IV

THE ORGANIC EFFECTS OF MUSIC

SECTION V

THE EFFECTS OF REPETITION AND FAMILIARITY

SECTION VI

THE EFFECTS OF MUSIC BESIDES AUDITORY AND ORGANIC

CHAPTER I

INTRODUCTION

W. V. Bingham

The studies of the effects of music presented in this volume have all been undertaken in the scientific spirit. The method of the laboratory and the tools of statistical procedure have been employed, yet not without the guiding insight of musician and æsthetician to furnish clues and to help in evaluating results. The contributors are not scientists only; they have also a competent acquaintance and a deep interest in the field of music whose secrets they are exploring.

The book is at once a response and a challenge. It is a response to the inquiry which any thoughtful listener makes, " What is this music doing to me ? " At the same time it is a challenge to science to explain more adequately than has as yet been done the nature and the mysteries of musical effects.

Just what does music do to us ? No comprehensive answer to this question could dispense with an analysis of the personal equation. How do we differ from one another in musical susceptibility ? What are the degrees of difference between people in their response to music and to particular sorts of music ? To what extent are these differences innate, a heritage from our differing ancestries ? To what extent are they traceable to environmental influences during infancy, childhood and youth ?

So fascinating an area of research would not have lain virtually unexplored throughout the years, were it not for the baffling complexity which it opposes to any scientific approach. The scientist prefers a problem with only one independent variable. He wants an experimental technique which rigidly controls every factor, unless it be the single one whose properties he is most interested in observing. But it is hard to make all the variables in a musical experiment stay put. We can control easily enough such complications as the time of day or the season of the year. We can control to our entire satisfaction the external conditions surrounding the listener, including not only the physical setting but also the social and the musical atmosphere in which a selection is heard. These, however, are after all relatively minor determiners of response. The two major determiners are the musical selection itself, on the one hand, and on the other, the listener. These two variable factors, which we may call the stimulus and the subject, are complex enough to challenge the best ingenuity of the experimenter.

Adequate control of the stimulus is virtually impossible without some such aid as the phonograph. How else can an investigator be certain that successive presentations of a musical stimulus are practically identical ? Musical science owes to Mr. Edison a great debt, for only by means of this, his favourite invention, can a song be repeated precisely and its effects measured. From the viewpoint of the experimenter, this value of the phonograph is comparable with its worth as a musical repository which preserves for later generations the renditions of supreme artists as well as the exotic melodies of vanishing savage tribes. The phonograph furnishes the means to control the musical stimulus and so makes more feasible a scientific study of musical effects.

The most baffling variable is the listener himself. How

is it possible to reach any generalizations regarding the effects of music so long as hearers differ greatly from each other in musical sophistication, in age and education, in personality and temperament, in musical ear and talent ?

We know that the same selection often affects two people differently. It may irritate one and soothe the other. It may hold Mrs. Smith's interest, while Smith is bored. One worker at a hand loom, whom I was observing, moved more rapidly and steadily while listening to jazz ; but another worker at the same time became so keyed-up that she tended repeatedly to exert too much pressure on reed, treadle, and shuttle, and, having to exercise more self-control to prevent errors, accomplished less than without the music. Her nervous system seemed to be at once more sensitive and less well organized than her companion's. The effect of the stimulus as measured by changes in amount of output was favourable in one case and unfavourable in the other because the listeners were different. Musical experimentation will always have this difficulty to face, because no two people are identical in their make-up.

The puzzle presented by this fact of wide variability in human nature is perhaps more baffling than at first appears, for a person changes even while listening to a musical selection. One can never experience a second time the precise sensations of a first hearing. The selection may be rendered just as it was before, but the listener can never again hear it with all the freshness of novelty. He has inevitably become modified by the first experience. With each repetition he is virtually a different listener.

But it is not necessary to be wholly daunted even by these complexities of human nature. Not alone in the realm of musical experience has science had to face and conquer these difficulties. All psychology has to reckon with individual differences. Biology has to study variations as well as types. The physiologist is not discouraged in his study of the effects of a certain diet because dyspeptics do not all respond to it alike ; he is sometimes content to know what reaction the food produces in a healthy person. The psychologist, too, seeks to learn the normal typical response to various kinds of music. He is doubly fortunate when in addition, he can formulate also, as some of the authors of this book have done, the laws governing the variations from this norm.

The contributions to musical science and psychological æsthetics which compose this volume are in the main chosen from among the papers submitted in a competition conducted by the American Psychological Association in 1921 for the most meritorious research on the effects of music. The funds for a prize of $500 were generously advanced by Mr. Thomas A. Edison, through the Edison-Carnegie Music Research, which the writer, with the assistance of Dr. Max Schoen and Dr. Esther L. Gatewood, was at the time conducting. The reports made by these investigators working in the psychological laboratory of the Carnegie Institute of Technology, although not submitted for consideration in connexion with the award of the prize, are in part included in this volume.

The investigations chosen for publication include experimental studies of the effects of stimulating and quieting music on heart action as measured by the Einthoven Galvanometer ; the effects of familiarity and repetition on affective response ; a comparison of reactions to classical and jazz selections ; types and modes of reaction to music ; the sensorial basis of music appreciation ; and individual differences in musical sensitivity.

The jury to select the most meritorious research consisted of Professor H. P. Weld, of Cornell, Professor H. D. Kitson, now of Columbia, and the writer. Consideration was given to each of the following points, the weight assigned to each point having previously been determined by a consensus of psychologists :—

> The problem : Its significance and relevance to the subject announced for the competition.
> Ingenuity and soundness of procedure adopted.
> Rigour of experimentation.
> Interpretation of results : analytical acumen ; rigour and coherence of argument.
> Presentation ; style.

Judged on such a basis, the choice rested on the admirably crisp and clear-cut report of experiments by Professor Margaret Floy Washburn and her student assistants at Vassar College. This prize-winning study on The Effects of Repetition is found on pages 199 to 210. It may well serve as a pattern for many future explorations in the domain of music psychology.

This competition was initiated by the writer because of a long-standing interest in the study of musical effects. It was nearly twenty years ago, in the psychological laboratories of Angell at Chicago and Münsterberg at Harvard that he sought to capture on the smoked surface of the kymographic drum those elusive changes in muscular tension which accompany the hearing of music.

The problem at that time was one of psychological æsthetics. What is a melody ? What makes out of one succession of tones a tune, while the same tones heard in a different order are not a tune but only a meaningless, formless jargon, devoid of interest or beauty ?

The experimental search for the bonds that tie together successive sounds and make out of a discrete series an æsthetic unity—a melody—led me to investigate the motor phenomena, the bodily movements, which consciously or unconsciously, every listener to a melody exhibits. Not every one taps his foot or sways his body to the rhythm of the music : but every listener who is at all musical, everyone to whom the succession of tones means anything, responds by exhibiting very slight but characteristic changes of muscular tonicity.

It is the listener, and not the performer alone, who creates the melody. In the act of response to the successive tones that strike upon his ear, he binds them together. If these tones are unrelated—incapable of stimulating a common motor response—they are of necessity apprehended as discrete, unmelodic. If, however, each tone initiates a response which is in effect a continuation of an act of adjustment already partially accomplished, it takes its place in a truly melodic series. And if the final tone is an end-tone, a tonic—if the response it provokes is the completion of the act for which the preceding adjustments have been a preparation—then the sounds are indeed perceived to form a unity, a melody.

To study these obscure but basic responses made by the organism I used as melodic stimuli only the simplest and briefest series of musical sounds : two successive tones, three, four, and at most seven. The complications of rhythm were rigidly excluded. Examination of the effects of these elementary melodic combinations was most illuminating. Out of the evidence came the hypothesis that the motor response of the listener is an essential determiner of melodic relationship between successive tones.

Emphasis was placed on the enormous importance of habituation and familiarity, and especially of the early musical environment in determining what tonal intervals a hearer perceives as related. Individual attitudes and the temporary mental set of the listener, also, were seen to have a share in explaining how particular melodic relationships come to be apprehended as they are. The listener's past and present, as well as the nature of the physical stimuli, help to make possible the interpretation of a succession of musical sounds as a melody. Quite recently this problem of melodic relationship and the nature of the tonic effect on which such investigations as Lipps, Stumpf, and, in this country, Max Meyer and the present writer had experimented has again been attacked by Paul Farnsworth, using as his materials the very shortest and simplest of melodies.

The studies in this volume, by way of contrast, deal for the most part with the effects of musical selections in their entirety. It is not the melodic fragment whose influence on the organism intrigues the interest of these investigators. It is the whole melody, heard in all the complex setting of its harmonic background. And it is not alone the motor phenomena induced by these melodies, but all their effects on feeling and thought as well as action, which form the objects of study.

Dr. Schoen has shouldered the burden of editing the several reports of investigation and weaving them into a sequence which gives the reader an excellent cross-section of contemporary inquiry into the problems of musical effects. To this task he brings the equipment of a psychologist who was first a violinist and later for several years a trainer of teachers of public school music. A pupil of Dr. C. E. Seashore, the dean of American investigators in the realm of music psychology, he has done much to spread among musicians an increased appreciation of the usefulness of the scientific method as an aid in appraising musical talent as well as in understanding the nature of musical effects.

Art and science are not intrinsically hostile. It is a

commonplace that many distinguished musicians—especially organists—have also been mathematicians. No one will deny that the thinker, and not alone the artist, is capable of appreciation. The æsthetic and the intellectual are equally valid modes in which to apprehend the values of experience. There is nothing inherently antagonistic between the love of beauty and the quest for truth.

This volume attests that at least one realm of æsthetic experience—the province of music and its effects is profitable and fascinating subject-matter for the research of the scientist as well as for the intuition of the artist or the meditation of the philosopher. Here, as in the sister arts of poetry, drama, painting, sculpture, and architecture, deeper insight and improved control may be expected when psychologists, with increased facilities and opportunities for research, bring to bear on problems of appreciation, taste and artistic creation the techniques of their young science.

SECTION I

TYPES OF LISTENERS TO MUSIC

Introductory Note.—That individuals vary enormously in their attitudes towards music—in what music means to them and in what they get out of it—is apparent to the most superficial observer. Even among the best and most cultivated minds in matters of art and literature extensive variations are found, from Johnson who found music to be " the costliest of rackets " to Carlyle to whom music was " a kind of inarticulate, unfathomable speech which leads us to the edge of the infinite, and lets us for moments gaze into that ". So widespread and evident is this variation that it has become proverbial, and conversations on " what is what " in music usually close with the ultimatum that " about tastes there is no disputing ".

Psychologically, this characteristic of human nature presents several problems, an adequate solution of which would have far-reaching educational value, in that it would cast some light upon the ever-present and complex question of aims and methods in music education. Some of these problems are (1) Are there any similarities in this apparent diversity of musical effects, similarities on the basis of which persons might be classified into types of listeners more or less distinct basically, and if so, what are the types and their distinguishing characteristics ? (2) To what are these differences due, to native endowment, or to training and experience, or to a combination of both ? (3) What are the relative æsthetic values of the diverse types of response, is any type more truly æsthetic than any one or all of the others ?

The two studies presented in this section deal directly with the first of these problems, and also have significant implications for the other questions. Professor Ortmann's approach is genetic. He shows how the attitude toward music develops, and how the individual differences arise in the course of this development, with suggestions as to the cause or causes for the origin of these variations. In contrast to Professor Ortmann's dynamic treatment, Professor Myers' treatment of the same problem is static, in that he classifies the mature, already formed, attitudes, and analyses and evaluates them.

It is noteworthy that the two studies, although approached from different angles, yet supplement each other in a striking and very suggestive manner.—EDITOR.

CHAPTER II

INDIVIDUAL DIFFERENCES IN LISTENING TO MUSIC

CHARLES S. MYERS

1. *Plan of the Investigation*

THIS study is based on the responses of fifteen persons to six musical compositions. These fifteen persons, nine men and six women, all university graduates or their wives, were in various degrees musical. Two of them, J. and M., were highly gifted professional musicians; three, B., F., and G., though not averse to music, may be regarded as relatively unmusical. Between these extremes are to be ranged three persons, H., K., and N., who were fairly accomplished amateur musicians; five, C., E., L., O., and P., who though unable to perform music, were of extremely artistic temperament; and two, A. and D., who may be described as possessing an average degree of musical taste. One of the listeners, E., was a Japanese. Eight of these persons served in a previous experiment conducted by the writer on individual differences of aspect adopted in listening to the tones of tuning-forks, simple and combined, presented singly and in pairs.[1]

In order to secure uniform presentation of the material, the phonograph was employed for the production of the music, using the best available records and instrument for the purpose. Most of the listeners found little difficulty in dismissing from their minds the artificial conditions of the experiment. They listened to the music as they would have listened to it in a concert hall. Indeed, one

---

[1] *British Journal of Psychology,* 1914, vii, 68–111.

person, C., of extremely artistic temperament though without musical training, remarked that the conditions were " ideal " for listening, as the comfort was greater than at a concert, and there were " no aggravating people and no worrying illumination ! "

The music consisted of Beethoven's Overture to Egmont (Op. 84), Tschaikowsky's Valse des Fleurs from his Casse Noisette Suite (Op. 71A), and his Italian Capriccio (Op. 45), Mendelssohn's Overture to the Hebrides (Fingal's Cave) (Op. 26), the first of Grieg's Symphonic Dances (Op. 64), and Kreisler's setting and playing of Couperin's Aubade Provencale—all save the last being orchestral performances.

Each person listened to two or three of these six records at a single sitting. More than one person never listened on any one occasion. Most of the listeners had two sittings, so that the average number of records to which each of them listened was between four and five. Before a person first listened at any sitting, he was always initially given a record to hear (not one of the above six), in order to become accustomed to the experimental conditions. He was seated in a comfortable armchair, with his back to the phonograph. The first time he heard any one of the six records, he was left absolutely free to relate his impressions and his attitudes at the close of it. He was then given pencil and paper and allowed to hear it a second time, noting down any further impressions in a mnemonic form, so that he would not fail to communicate them to me at the close of the second hearing and could describe how that hearing differed from the first. By a simple arrangement of a travelling index, and a fixed scale which was attached to the instrument, any required part of the pieces could be reproduced from the record at will. With the help of this contrivance, certain selected short passages were finally presented to the listener and he was asked to record his impressions of them.

2. Comparison with the Results of the Writer's previous Investigation

In all those persons who had previously submitted to introspection in the tuning-fork experiments, it was easy to recognize broadly the same aspects as they had there displayed when they came to listen to the more complex material of a musical work. That is to say, the material might appeal to them (1) for the sensory emotional or conative experience which it aroused ; (2) for the associations which it suggested, (3) for its use or value considered as an object, or (4) for its character personified as a subject. These four aspects, which were previously distinguished respectively as (1) the intra-subjective, (2) the associative, (3) the objective, and (4) the character, were readily recognizable, more or less according to the prominence they had exhibited in the introductory, more elementary tonal experiments. Thus one person, A., of average musical taste, who, when listening to tones, had proved predominantly of the associative type, recorded such associations as the following when listening to the music : " I was in the Queen's Hall, a fair girl in a pink dress was playing and another girl was accompanying her. The violinist had a sad look about her. I felt she had had a sorrow in her life." " I saw F— playing it as a duet as he used to do." " It started with a stage full of people : a tremendous lot of movement about it and brightness. The people were all in costumes. Then a singer came on from a house on the right side of the stage, telling a pathetic love-story. Then I lost the solo part, the stage became dark, and all the people left, except, I believe, the singer who remained in some quiet corner." " It reminds me of Ely Cathedral." Compare these statements with this person's previous replies when a series of pure tones was given her : " I saw a woman in evening dress as if she were singing." " I saw a certain room with F— at the instrument just starting to play with his right hand." " I think I saw the inside of a church." Or take another listener, G., relatively unmusical, who when confronted with single tones had always shown a keen conative tendency ; a strong desire to do something with them, e.g. : " I tried to connect it with piano sounds but couldn't." " I can't join it on to piano sounds : I try to imagine it in its place in a piece played by a pianola." " It made me wonder whether it was a sound that could come into a tune." " I considered what was the difference between this and the last." He is always trying to give the tone utilitarian value. When listening to the phono-graph records he proved to be one of the few who were preoccupied with drawbacks of the instrument. " I don't like it. It's the fault of the phonograph—its tinny sound. . . Then I liked it, but my mind was much occupied trying to pick out the instruments of the orchestra. It seemed to me as if certain instruments felt the ill-effects of the phonograph . . . more than others." " I did not seem able to keep up with the more excited mood, and I had a feeling of disappointment at this inability." Another listener, C., who in the case of the tuning-fork experiments, had referred frequently to the " movement " which the sound underwent, when his attention was directed from one tone to the next, constantly alluded to the " patterns " formed by the music in the present experiments. " It falls into a pattern." " It is the sequence of sounds of different pitch that makes the pattern." " Then the pattern changed." " Then came a pattern of different type."

Here is an example of a listener, D., who in the earlier experiments with tuning-fork tones had shown herself to belong to the physiological sub-group of the intra-subjective aspect, returning such answers as " I felt a touch on the tympanum " ; " I felt a stinging up the right arm, as if the first finger touched a copper spring that rebounded " ; " I felt warm in the ear " ; " I had a lazy feeling." Following are some extracts from her reports on the phonograph pieces : " A restful feeling throughout . . . like one of going downstream while swimming . . . I wanted to throw myself back and be carried along." " During the dance movement I imaged a gentle breeze and felt diaphanous things floating in the wind . . . The breeze came in contact with my right cheek." " Suddenly it seemed as if the orchestra was in a pavilion in a garden, which then revived all kinds of organic sensations ; walking about in the garden, feeling warm. Then I realized that I had been warm before." " My two ears seemed joined together, drawn to one another by something elastic." " An echo heard after each chord, with definite vibration inside the right ear." " A very definite olfactory sensation of open air and grass." In the tuning-fork experiments this person had shown tendencies also to the character type and to visual symbolism, describing, for example, a given sound " as purple and maroon, which are ' like the lights one feels rather than sees ', as in shutting the eyes in a bright light or in pressing on the closed eyelids. There is no outline or demarcation between the purple and maroon. They seem to fill the entire field ". [1] So, too, in listening to music, she reports : " Flourishes, flamboyant architecture, suggested." " A ball raised by something elastic and falling back by its own weight : this happened three or

[1] Op. cit., 84, 85.

four times." " The piece seemed represented by long and short dashes. No sense of extent, no feeling of areas— only contrast by dashes."

It is, I think, of no little psychological and experimental interest to note the consequent value of investigations with the simplest materials for our understanding of the aspects adopted, the kind of appeal made, in the case of works of art. It seems probable that the experience of beauty is rooted in man's remote past when it could be evoked by such simple material as one or two tones or splashes of colour, i.e. by the most primitive forms conceivable of art material, just as to-day it is evoked by more complex forms.

3. *Comparison with the Results of previous Investigation on Colours*

But there are exceptions to the general correspondence between the aspects of listening to tones and of regarding colours.[1] In the case of A., for example, who proved to be strongly of the associative type for tones and music, " a colour is almost a human being and is endowed with such personal attributes as morose, cheerful, insincere, serious, playful, etc." When, however, she comes to listen to music, this character aspect, though by no means abolished, is largely replaced by the intra-subjective aspect—i.e. the sensory effects, the changes in feeling, the experiences of self-activity obtained from the music. She reports, " That was lovely . . . Something lifting, raising you inside. Like what one gets in church." " I imagine I am going to die, as if life were just ebbing out." " A great feeling of happiness ; followed by expansion inside, leading to great excitement and breathlessness for a moment." Nevertheless, the character aspect may

[1] Op. cit., 86–90.

be detected : e.g. " Very, very beautiful, but very mournful and sad : a drawing out of the agony." " It tried to
be light-hearted, but was all the time very sad." " The
first two bars are like feelings of anticipation, then that
lovely feeling of depth and goodness coming out of you
that you get in church. Yet all through, very very sad.
Sensations of something coming up from the abdomen
and surging up to the head." " I cannot get anything out
of it but depression. A delightful feeling of welcoming
the end . . . I had feelings of sorrow and dissatisfaction
with everything. They gained on me. All the time I was
trying to get the better of those feelings, but they wouldn't
leave me." We see here how the character aspect may be
inhibited and replaced by the intra-subjective aspect,
i.e. by the strong feelings to which in this subject the
music gives rise. In the case of the present study, the
multiplicity of attitudes increases still further. Hardly
any listener shows himself absolutely pure to one type,
to the complete exclusion of others. The material here
is far more complex, comprising no longer merely pure
tones, but also melody, rhythm, tone colour, polyphony,
harmony, etc. Even in the simple experiments with tuning-
fork tones there were indications that, whereas the liking
or disliking of a *single* tone was determined more often
by *sensual* changes, in the case of two simultaneous tones
it was determined rather by emotional and conative
changes. Moreover, unlike a tone, a colour, or a picture,
a musical composition is not presented all at once as a
whole, but is unfolded gradually, like a poem or drama.
Such differences in complexity and in mode of presentation
will naturally result in a many-sided appeal to the person's
possible aspects, now inviting one, now another, now a
third, whereas in the case of the more abstract, simpler
material and with less natural, more restricted methods of

procedure, fewer aspects are appealed to, and of these only the more habitual and the more ready.

From these considerations we should expect to find that different kinds of music may evoke different aspects in the same listener, so that he comes to realize that there are many different ways in which he can appreciate music. As one of my listeners remarked, " Sometimes I listen to music seeing the orchestra and attending to the *technique*, sometimes enjoying visions of forests, etc., that come before me, sometimes paying regard to the meaning, the sadness, etc., of the piece."

An artificial purity of type may arise from the process, conscious or unconscious, of inhibition. We have seen, for example, how the character aspect may be inhibited by the intra-subjective aspect : instead of regarding the music as a personality, the listener's attention is directed to the sensations, emotions and impulses evoked in him. Here a ' higher ' aspect is replaced by a ' lower ' (for aesthetically the character aspect stands unquestionably higher than the intra-subjective). But the converse may also occur. Instead of the lower aspect being released, it may be controlled by higher inhibition. One of my listeners observed, " I should have felt distinctly wretched . . . I very nearly let myself go." Such higher control is especially exercised over the associative aspect. " I object to these suggestions (i.e. associations)," says another ; " for I find then that the music . . . is not listened to for itself. I want to do that." " If I had not had to give introspective data," says yet another, " probably the images would have passed unnoticed."

4. *The Objective Aspect in the Technician*

It is interesting to find that the objective aspect, in which the musical material is considered in reference to the listener's standard, occurs most frequently among those technically trained in music, who tend to adopt a critical attitude and are interested in the material of their art. Consider, for example, the reports of the professional musical listener, M. : " I noticed the second horn was too loud . . . When the second tune came with the 'cellos, it didn't stand out enough." " I noticed by what simple means in these modern days he gets his effects . . . I noticed also . . . how he gathered up his climax by syncopation." " As always in Beethoven, one must notice the tremendous . . . contrasts, especially dynamic contrasts. His crescendos always gives me pleasure. Beethoven makes scale passages so much more interesting than, say, Liszt." " As usual, the violinist uses too much *vibrato* . . . The sweep up the strings made me feel quite sick." This person remarked, " I now nearly always view music from the critical standpoint. I conduct ; I compose. I always want to know how the conductor is getting effects if it is a *new* work, and what will be his rendering if it is an old one . . . I never think of ' programme ' unless it is suggested to me. . . To me music is never sad or joyful. I only get æsthetic impression."

This highly musical person believes, then, that in listening to music he suppresses not merely the more lowly intra-subjective and associative aspects, not merely all personal feelings, activities and imaginations, but also the character aspect, in favour of the objective aspect, the critical, analytical standpoint. Now it is interesting to find that this very person, when he was presented in the experiments with tuning-fork tones, had shown very distinctly the character aspect, personifying tones as " trivial ", " grim ", " mysterious ", " stupid ", " silly ", " bony ", " bare ". Even in the present musical experiments, a tendency towards the same aspect is revealed. " The cadenzas," he remarks, " are rather vulgar and horrid." " That is simply a piece of empty pomposity, holding you up to expect something beautiful, and then you get *that*." " The introductory solo accompaniment . . . is in the last degree trivial."

Upon the release of the character aspect even the associative aspect occasionally escapes in this listener from its inhibition. Thus the trivial character of the music suggests to him the stage. " I saw the orchestra and footlights." The same escape of associations had occurred when he was listening to the tuning-fork tones : a " stupid " note suggesting " a stupid parrot ", and a " materialistic " tone, suggesting a successful tradesman. These associations seemed to be determined exclusively by recent experience. Thus the stupid parrot was connected with a recent visit to the " Zoo ". The stage music, just mentioned, " carried me back to the time I heard the opening of Rimsky-Korsakow's opera, *Ivan the Terrible*, last night." So, too, his recognition of the Hebrides Overture brought up visual images of " a cave, rocks, seawaves . . . a sea serpent poking its head out of the cave (suggested by the trombones), dancing spray, with the sun on it. " I could draw the exact picture. I have been reading lately about Hebridean folk songs."

The occurrence of these associations filled M. with amazement. " It is not like me at all," he protests. On another occasion he observes, " I opened this with a dog fight. . . The opening of the second part was a dance of savages ; (this is *amazing* to me) I could see the red and blue round the loin cloths. Then, I think, I pulled myself together." In other words, he checked or inhibited all tendency to association, which under these experimental conditions was specially favoured. Another listener, D., emphatically of the intra-subjective type, similarly remarked, " I always try and banish all imagination when listening to music." What a contrast this presents to the highly artistic, but musically untrained listener, P., who insists, " Music always gives me the sight of so many charming things. That's why I like listening to it."

Trivial, unreal, or meretricious music is specially liable to evoke in imagination stage scenery, the hearer regarding the feelings or actions of the persons imaged from a distance without sharing himself in them. " I was up in the theatre," reports K., " looking down." " *I*," reports E., " felt no deep emotion. But there was much emotion in *the* soldiers." " The beginning," says L., " reminded me of a stage, people coming on. It was trivial, theatrical." Observe now the contrast. " Then it passes to out-of-doors, real, not stage-like, in a wood, with sunlight, a vast procession of people slowly moving, . . . with gold-coloured dresses, some green, all brilliant."

5. *The Absence of Associations in the Most Unmusical*

It would be indeed surprising if the tendency to associations were lacking in the most musical persons. For in all the rest of the listeners associations are present in a varying degree, save in C., who is ever occupied with his " patterns " and F. and G., the two most unmusical. Both the two latter adopt predominantly the intra-subjective aspect. F. allows the sounds to act physiologically upon him, and it is only as a *pis aller* that he advances reasons for his preferences from the objective

aspect. He does not " trouble about the meaning "
of music, probably because it has none consciously
for him (musically or otherwise). He never attends
concerts. He hardly knows one tune from another.
The following are samples of his reports :—" It's just
the kind of thing I like. But . . . why I like it, I can't
see. . . I didn't like the beginning when the high notes
came. I never can stand high-pitched notes . . . (Here
he is driven to the objective aspect) . . . I always like a
thing of low intensity, gentle : that, I feel, is a much
better kind of thing than a good crash of sound . . . I was
soothed almost as if asleep . . . Very charming indeed.
Just the kind of thing I like . . . I can't think of any
meaning of the slow and the quick themes . . . I shouldn't
trouble about the meaning." Despite the fact that he is
extremely unmusical and gets so little æsthetic enjoyment from music, F. shows almost invariable correct
taste in his judgment of good and bad music.

The absence of associations in the two most unmusical
persons is of undoubted interest in regard to the origin
and fundamental basis of musical enjoyment. The
influence of sexual experience and of juvenile imagination
is shown in the fact that the commonest figures evoked
in the recorded associations were those of lovers, dancers,
soldiers, villagers, savages, fairies, fauns, and goblins.
Associations of sexual character occurred in eight of the
fifteen listeners (C., E., F., H., J., K., L., O.) and
associations of dancing in ten (A., D., E., H., J., K.,
L. M., O., P.). Six persons (A., B., J., K., M., P.)
reported associations in which a stage full of moving
people was presented ; six (D., H., E., L., O., P.) in
which the scene was laid in the open air ; and five
(A., B., D., M., P.) in which the orchestra, the conductor,
or a musical instrument appeared. Three persons

(A., H., K.) imagined themselves in a concert hall;
three (A., H., O.) in church.

There can be no doubt that such associations were
often responsible for the æsthetic enjoyment of the
music in these experiments. Indeed, the close biological
relation of the origin of music to sexual display and to
movements of the body in dancing would have made
this conclusion *a priori* probable. In the grossly
unmusical, music evokes no associations, because it
evokes no corresponding emotion. In the professional
musician, music also evokes few or no associations,
because he tends to inhibit them by his assumption
of a critical, objective attitude. Among the most
highly musical associations tend also to be repressed,
because the music comes to be listened to for its own
meaning and beauty, apart from the meaning and beauty
derived from associations. In four of the five persons
whose temperament was extremely artistic but who had
little or no technical knowledge of music, associations
were to a large extent replaced by symbols, e.g. of pattern,
colour, or expanse, the activities of which, however,
tended themselves to evoke associations.

6. *The Occurrence of Associations among the Musical*

When the average person listens to music, then,
associations are enjoyed for their own sake, adding
enormously to the total æsthetic appreciation obtainable.
The associations may be in themselves beautiful: they
invite the listener to share in the beauty of a story and
in the emotions of the persons created in his imagination.
Among the more highly musical I find that associations
are more particularly apt to intrude when the music
is felt to be "stagey", unreal, meretricious, or vulgar.
Thus M. reports associations as the music "began to

get more barbaric " and as he " lost interest in the music ". He observes, however, " the middle of the second movement (which he enjoyed) switched me off my imagery, and I returned to the pure consideration of the music."

It is by no means strange that associations should appear among the highly musical when music lacks interest or inherent beauty, whereas the less musical tend to appreciate music not so much on the grounds of its inherent beauty as for the enjoyment of the associations evoked. The explanation depends on difference of æsthetic level, the level of the musically gifted person standing higher than that of one averagely musical. So long as the former attending merely to the music, *qua* music, can maintain his high level of æsthetic enjoyment, associations are debarred from consciousness. But when for any reason he fails to maintain that level, e.g. because his æsthetic appreciation ceases, then the products of lower-level aspects enter, e.g. associations more or less incongruous with the enjoyment of beauty.

In order that associations may be enjoyed for their beauty, either the music must be wholly neglected, and the story, the imagery, the wealth of colour enjoyed as if it were a work of art—which is seldom possible—or the associations must blend or fuse in their general meaning (on which their beauty depends) with that of the music. Otherwise they can have no *æsthetic* value, but are merely effectively toned with pleasure or displeasure, or at most excite in the listener feelings of joy or distress, according to their cognitive or emotional content. In the following report from one of the listeners we see the distinction between unfused associations and associations of actively æsthetic value which fuse with that of the music.

" I object to these suggestions, for I find that the music
. . . is not listened to for itself. But," he continues,
" when the suggestions and the music absolutely blend,
there is the completest and greatest enjoyment, greater
than when there is music alone. They won't blend
here, because the dramatic scene will go on quite well,
independently of the music."

To quote another example of this lack of fusion,
" It produced," says D., " the idea of someone trying
to be persuasive. I wanted to know how the persuasive-
ness would go on . . . if it would succeed. . . It seemed to
be a dramatic development without any images. This
dramatic is quite distinct from the musical development.
They run parallel. There are two people concerned
in the dramatic development—the persuader and the
persuaded. . . There is no response to the persuasion :
it is a failure. The characters disappear ; and the music
behaves like a Greek chorus, going over what has occurred
in a philosophical manner." Fusion appears to be
here lacking between the wordless meaning of the music
and the meaning of the imageless thoughts it evoked.

7. *The Relation of the Character Aspect to the Intra-
subjective Aspect*

Is the character aspect towards music derived from
the intra-subjective or is it independent of it ? That
the character aspect is of higher æsthetic value than the
intra-subjective is fairly certain. But the relationship
between the two presents an interesting problem.

In the experiments with tuning-fork tones, it was
found that such characters as " jolly ", or " high-spirited "
may be ascribed to a sound or a colour even under conditions when the person himself feels sad or depressed.
As a further proof of the independence of the

" characterization " of music of the intra-subjective experience to which the music gives rise, the following reports may be quoted. A. : " The piece sounded cheerful in certain parts. But I felt in a contrary grain all the time." N. : ' It's all so intensely sad. All the time I was wondering whether it was cheap or not. I came to the conclusion that I ought to be moved. I *was much* moved by it after this conclusion. It was quite upsetting ; it made me feel sad. I still see the long funeral procession." That is to say, the sadness of the listener was secondary to the sadness characterized in the music. So, too, another subject remarked, " I noticed first the mournfulness of the music and then its effect on me." Or N. : " A distinctly pathetic ring about it. I should have felt distinctly wretched if I had got regularly into it, but I keep myself from this at a concert. I very rarely let myself go." Or J. : " There was a note of sadness among the dancers in parts, a sort of regretfulness. I think this sadness affected me secondarily to the stage sadness." Or H. : " The music seemed as if it were joking with me : it made me want to smile."

We see then that the art material may be personalized and characterized as morbid, jovial, insincere, dainty, mystic, reckless, playful, etc., without necessarily having previously evoked, or consequently evoking morbid, jovial, etc., feelings in the listener. The varying degree in which the listener may identify himself with the character ascribed by him to the music, is well illustrated by the following reports :—H. : " I felt the yearning character of the first motif," " a sense of tears in it— which was partly in the *motif* and partly in *me*." " It reminded me of a time when I actually wept in listening to an intensely beautiful chorus, so beautiful that it hurt." Q. : " It has expressions rather in the way that a face has expressions. I didn't see a face . . . I almost personified the music as having expression, a shade of feeling being implied." " There is something sinister about it. It gave me a feeling that made me appreciate how sinister it was."

We have to remember that a tendency to personify inanimate objects is extremely primitive and deep-rooted. As Stout remarks,[1] " The cataract or the whirl-pool appears a living thing to the poet in his poetic moods : for in these moods he ignores the fact that the water is behaving in accordance with certain abstract laws under certain given conditions. This fact is not *ignored* by the savage : it has never been realized by him. Hence what may be called a transcient play of imagination in the civilized mind is the permanent and serious attitude of the savage mind." If Stout had at his own disposal a more strongly developed character aspect, he would realize that it is the persistence of this so-called mark of the savage that leads to the æsthetic personalization of colours, tones, and music.

Now it is evident that for æsthetic enjoyment to be perfect there must be no conflict between the feelings of the listener himself and those inherent in the character of the music. Nor must there be conflict between the character of the music and that of the persons or the story which the listener's imagination may call forth. The need for harmony between these three factors— the feelings of the listener, those inherent in the character of the music, and those of the persons in the story imagined—is well illustrated in the following report from one of the listeners. O. : " I almost personified the music . . . a shade of feeling being implied. I felt

[1] *Manual of Psychology*, 3rd ed., 685.

that I had had that feeling before and could sympathize with what the chap was trying to explain." Such sympathy and understanding must add as much to the conditions favouring æsthetic appreciation as antipathy and ignorance must militate against them. E.g. A. : " The piece sounded cheerful in certain parts. But I felt in a contrary grain all the time." Or " I don't know what the end was . . . I couldn't fit it into my lines of thought." Or G. : " I couldn't keep up with the more excited mood and was hence disappointed."

8. *Symbolization of the Art Material*

In some persons, as we have seen, instead of the music being endowed with the characters of a human personality, it is symbolized in material form, e.g. by dashes, prisms, cylinders, circles, and patterns. D. : " The piece seemed represented by long and short dashes. No sense of extent, no feeling of areas—only contrast by dashes." C. : " A frightfully interesting medley of sounds from the pattern point of view." " The pattern is perhaps most like those of glass marbles. It is in three dimensions. Up and down, right and left, for progress of melody and thirdly, depth, i.e. volume." " Then the pattern changed : the strands separated out, the lower patterns accentuated, the upper rippling." " Then came a pattern of a different type, beginning with zig-zags, obliquely transverse strands from lower left to upper right, going through a horizontally moving pattern." " I saw a frame," reports P., " containing a spiral growing larger and smaller. . . The spiral rotated : it had different coloured strands. The frame widened and narrowed, as the spiral changed in size." There is obviously a close analogy between the rise and fall of pitch, the blending, interweaving, and segregation of different simultaneous themes, the motor effects of various rhythms and syncopations on the one hand, and the forms and movements of geometrical designs, on the other.

Such tendency to ascribe form and movement to a series of sounds is doubtless related to the not uncommon endowment of sounds with colour ; one tone, one tone quality, one key, one word or letter or vowel appearing of one colour, another of another colour. The actual colour is in part, though probably not wholly, determined by early, long-forgotten, perhaps for some reason repressed, experiences. But the tendency for such coloured hearing runs in families : it is inherited, not acquired. Such colours appear in actual visual imagery occasionally in the replies of the listeners. Thus P. reports : " At the pause I see a space, a grey misty space, clean-cut at each end, extending from left to right. This visual part is there all the time but it outlasts the auditory " : i.e. when the music pauses the colour continues. Colours may be suggested not by the sounds alone but by the associations to which the music gives rise, and they may in turn suggest other associations. Thus, the just-mentioned " grey " arose, explains P., because the music " reminds me of dawn-grey, fresh and nice ". And having obtained the " lovely grey ", " I then saw a frieze, not a real good Greek one, but a Thorwaldsen or a Canova frieze."

" Following the pattern," says C., " is my greatest enjoyment in music. If I cannot follow it, I lose the beauty : I lose my bearings. There is no longer meaning in its movement. Right or left in the pattern may be compared to the behindness of the past. When the pattern is absent, the beauty lies in its clear-cut character of gloom, menace, and languor and simplicity." " I am now able to distinguish the parts of the individual movements. This enhances my enjoyment. I am able to follow it better. It makes the pattern clearer." He says that he tends to move with the pattern and is willing finally to surrender himself to it. Apparently his intra-subjective experience is helped by the pattern to the full appreciation and to the æsthetic enjoyment of the music. The music, then, appears to him in a form midway between a living person and a mechanical object. But when he can get no patterns of rhythmic or polyphonic foundation to enjoy, when, e.g. he listens to a simple melody or to a single tone, the character aspect comes to the fore with such descriptions as " plaintive ", " poignant ", " child-like ", " wailing ". " I might," he explains, " cry out at any moment, not from pain or sorrow. On the contrary, I enjoy it." It would appear as if the pattern or other symbolic figure was a half-way elaboration of the object-matter, not reaching to the height and the free organic independence of the character aspect, but kept low by the trammels of association and intra-subjective factors.

9. *The Æsthetic Value of the Pragmatic and Objective Aspects*

The purely pragmatic and objective aspects in which the art material is considered in relation to its use and to the person's standard of values are in themselves incapable of inducing the æsthetic experience. But they are indirectly of great importance. For the conception of a standard, although it cannot induce the experience of the beautiful, is of obvious use in forming a judgment of its æsthetic value. Thus we found that F., despite the scant æsthetic enjoyment he derived from music, invariably showed himself correct in his judgment between good and bad music. To treat the art material as a mere inanimate object having a certain value on reference to the person's standard, is, as we have seen, merely a last resource in the case of the untrained ; while in the case of the technician, it is the consequence of his absorption in the material. It is the refuge of the untrained in the absence of the potentially æsthetic aspects of character, association, and intra-subjective experience. It is the resource of the artist, in his endeavour by repression to escape from the influence of the other aspects, in order, it may be, to attain the highest appreciable beauty of music, the beauty of musical meaning which is inexpressible in any other terms.

The pragmatic aspect may have considerable æsthetic value by entering into combination with the other aspects. The use of material may readily evoke the intra-subjective attitude ; the appreciation of the *import* of the art object being followed by, say, impulses to do something with it, or by sensory or emotional changes in the subject, all of which may come to have æsthetic significance. Lastly, the personifying process, seen in its full development in the character aspect, may invest the changing melodic, rhythmic, and harmonic forms, as we have shown, with a *quasi*-animate activity, e.g. of moving patterns or forms which may enhance the æsthetic enjoyment of the music.

10.   *The Æsthetic Value of the Intra-Subjective Aspect*

Meaning of some sort, of course, there must be for the experience of beauty, and the lowest form of meaning which any stimulus takes is just the sensations which it directly evokes in us. Thus the lowest kind of beauty is experienced when the person adopts purely the intra-subjective attitude, surrendering himself to the sensory, emotional, and impulsive effects of the music. So long, however, as the listener gives himself up to the enjoyment of such experiences, all that he gets is delight or joy, not beauty. As Bullough rightly points out,[1] a process of psychical " distancing " is required in order that any of his sensations or emotions may appear beautiful. One must look on them with a certain detachment, to a certain extent impersonally. He has to project the beauty into his sensory, emotional, or conative experience, instead of subjectively appreciating the delight or joy to which they give rise. He has to look on them as a spectator, and in some measure at least to regard that experience as constituting in and for itself a living, unitary, independent entity.

Next, in order of development, to enjoying his own feelings, comes the listener's submission to following the enjoyment of the feelings of others, e.g. of the imagined performers, or, in the case of the character aspect, of the music itself. With this must develop a sympathy, more or less perfect, with the experiences he is following, e.g. one of my listeners, E., reports : " I cannot feel emotion in listening to music, unless I feel that I am moving in the same emotional attitude as the persons (imaged)." And B. observes : " Then a long pause which seemed annoyed and confused. I participated in the annoyance and confusion. Then a revolt. Then once again he subdued them. Peace and triumph seemed to reign. . . But I had no feeling in myself of success."

How frequently the person tends to identify his feelings with those of the creatures of his imagination, while listening to music, is well illustrated by the following quotations. J. : " I got the impression of people dancing,

---

[1] *British Journal of Psychol.*, 1912, v, 87–118.

I think, on the stage. I saw the moving figures—young people of both sexes. It struck me as a representation of a dance in the open air. There was a note of sadness among the dancers, a sort of regretfulness. I think that the sadness affected me and came secondarily to the stage sadness." Or again : " I saw one person alone to start with, asking for or expecting others to come and gradually a great crowd came running towards him. I distinctly felt I wanted to move with them."

Complete surrender may induce a state of transport or ecstasy. My Japanese listener E. reports : " Sometimes I lose myself in the music. . . I am unconscious and forgetful of myself." Another, K., reports : " I felt the effect of being carried away, partly emotional, partly strain and tenseness of body." But the surrender must be under voluntary control, or, as another of the hearers says : " I distrust them (the noisy parts) rather as an attempt to carry me away by mere force."

Complete surrender is incompatible with æsthetic enjoyment. This, as we have already suggested, depends on a certain detachment of the art material from one's Self, so that the object is judged to be itself beautiful. That beauty may be attached to sensations, feelings, etc., is indicated by the following extracts from the notes of E. : " The special feeling I get from music makes it beautiful. It gives me a tender poetic feeling, almost pity." Or as another, H., explains : " Certain short phrases gave me quite a beautiful thrill, localized in the diaphragm—like the feeling that early morning brightness gives one." When those feelings are re-garded as living entities from the standpoint of an onlooker, they may be deemed beautiful as objects of experience.

11. *The Æsthetic Value of the Meaning of Music*

So, too, the beauty of music may be derived from the story it suggests. " There she is," says P., " the little fairy. A sentimental sort of pantomime for children. . . Children dancing—not grown-ups. . . Man dressed in red with feather plumes. Don't you see the fairies ? Yes. It's a sylvan sort of thing." No wonder that she asserts, " Music always gives me the sight of so many charming things. That's why I like listening to it." " I generally try," says E. similarly, " to make a story out of a piece."

The meaning of the music may be also expressed more generally, with reference to our affective " attitudes ". Thus B. reports : " An insistent questioning and perhaps an unsatisfactory reply. . . A muffled knock which is disregarded. Then it took more definitely the form of someone's conscience being appealed to in vain. . . It came in words ' You know you should '. Then with ' Can't you see I can't do it ? ' All quite impersonal. The man had yielded to the temptation, but had not succeeded in quelling his conscience. Still the voice of menace came pricking out during the enjoyment."

We have already alluded to the need for appreciating sincerity and genuineness in music. An illustration may be quoted from O., who remarks, " . . . in the middle its expression changed to being true to life, real stuff, though I did not fully understand it." And from E., " I felt that there was no reality in it. It was a mere mechanical imitation . . . like a painting imitating a great master."

The importance of finding one or other of such meanings, before æsthetic experience is possible for some persons, is exemplified by such reports as B. : " No central idea in it. Never knew where I was " ; and E. : " Too much bothered about finding meaning to be able to see any beauty." In default of any other meaning, a subject is liable to revert to the more primitive forms of the imagination. "The whole," says one listener, "has no meaning in the least to me. I don't understand it. I am catching hold of any image I can get."

The more completely the meaning is concerned with the listener's notions of utility, the more impossible is it *per se* to get æsthetic appreciation. Whether we consider an art object well or ill-fitted to express its purpose, will not determine in us an experience of beauty. If we find it ill-fitted, this will debar us from readily experiencing beauty in it. If we find it well-fitted to express its purpose, our experience of beauty may be enhanced by our admiration and wonder. But the realization of appropriateness or perfection alone will not suffice to evoke an æsthetic experience. Nor will the mere following of analysis and appreciation of musical form. The object of beauty must be regarded not as a satisfactory piece of man-made mechanism, but as a living organic whole, without direct reference to our own value and use of it.

But there is always a meaning in music, apart from what may be obtained from feelings, stories, actions, colours, patterns, and language. Recognition of this fact becomes clearer with the development of musical appreciation. "When I see the pictures (the images evoked) they take up almost all my attention," protests M., "so that I have the feeling 'Dear me! I'm not listening', and then I get back to the music." So too, C., objects: "I cannot . . . conceive music *saying* anything," and another, H., explains: "Music has a meaning, but always in musical tones. I couldn't put it into words. It always irritates me to be asked to do this."

It is clear that when there is a possibility of so many different sources of meaning, some present in consciousness, other inhibited, but each tending to some particular response on the part of the listener, there must be a general harmony between these various meanings for æsthetic enjoyment to reach its climax. Likewise there must arise the ability to grasp the musical piece as a whole. Whereas painting is presented in space, music is presented in time. Whereas we seldom find that parts of a painting are beautiful, in music we are apt to get æsthetic experience here and there ; and it is only after the highest flight of synthesis that we can find enjoyment in the beauty of the music as a whole. " I felt," says H., " the whole piece as one. I felt the player conceived it as a whole." " This part," says another, K., " jarred and worried me, because it didn't seem to fit in with the other." A third listener complains, " I haven't grasped it as a whole." " Not an artistic whole," is the criticism of a fourth listener, J. " I thought," says yet another, " of the general shape and balance of the whole. . . I liked the contrast of the two sections." " Making notes," objects D., " made me only see the piece in bits."

12. *The Importance of Distance*

We can see now how the various aspects which we have distinguished in the listener may each play a part in the awareness of beauty, and how the different fundamental connexions of music, with courtship, with dancing, and with rudimentary language, may each contribute to æsthetic enjoyment. These different connexions may be differently stressed in different persons to-day, so that one tends specially to sexual, another to dramatic, another to verbal associations with music. But we come to recognize that, apart from these connexions, music may be appreciated for its own inherent beauty, that is to say, apart from its sensuous, emotional or conative influences and from associations, symbols, and products of "animistic" characterizations. The one common and essential attitude required for æsthetic enjoyment is one of detachment. The listener must view the music, as Bullough rightly insists, from a certain psychical "distance". If that distance be excessive, as occurs in listening for the first time to exotic music or to other unfamiliar styles of music, the person feels too remote to get, as it were, to grips with the art material. It is over-distanced. On the other hand, it is under-distanced, when he surrenders himself wholly to its influence in such a way that he is a more or less passive instrument played upon by the music, without paying any regard to his sensations, images, emotions, or impulses, save in so far as they have immediately personal and "practical" import.

13. *The Importance of the "Mystic" Feeling*

There are three main lines of activity which take us away from the purely practical, everyday aspect of our experiences. The simplest and most primitive is play. This fundamentally consists in giving a fictitious value to our motor behaviour. The second is phantasy, in which, as in day-dreaming, wrapped up in our Selves, we allow our imagination full play, regardless of the realities of our environment. The third consists in mystical experience in which we lose the normal awareness of our own individuality, and of its relation to our surroundings. The ecstasies (active and passive) of love and religion afford the most striking and undoubted instances of this kind of experience—the lost relation of the Self to its environment. I believe that our experience of beauty always partakes in some degree of this mystical or ecstatic character. Nowhere in art or nature as in music do we more keenly feel this " uplifting of the soul " as we term it, or as we may come to term it, this " uplifting of the unconscious ". But the mystical or ecstatic feeling must not be allowed to go too far ; otherwise we are carried away beyond our ability to experience beauty. On the other hand, unless we do, in however small degree, surrender our practical, everyday attitude that defines the relation of ourselves to our environment, unless we feel ourselves in that mysterious poetical atmosphere, I do not believe that beauty can be experienced, whether in music, painting, sculpture, architecture, or dancing ; whether in imagination, in a mathematical problem or in a purely sensory or emotional experience.

CHAPTER III

TYPES OF LISTENERS.   GENETIC CONSIDERATIONS

OTTO ORTMANN

THE problem of analyzing and classifying responses to music into types, is at the same time intensely interesting and notoriously difficult. It is interesting because every concert-goer has had, at one time or another, personal experience with it ; and it is difficult because of the immensely complex nature of the human organism. The history of the problem is rich in incoördinated data, poor in clear-cut conclusions. This is to be expected from the nature of the case. For we cannot well separate the problem of musical enjoyment from some treatment of general æsthetics, attributes of sensation, psychology of rhythm, harmony, melody; physiology, and numerous other phases, an inclusion of which would extend our treatment to the dimensions of a comprehensive general psychology of music, and an exclusion of which condenses the treatment to a necessarily fragmentary and somewhat inconclusive presentation. The former is impossible here, the latter inadvisable. Accordingly, a middle course is followed in this study. The readiness with which concrete examples of different kinds of response to music can be gathered, and the adaptability of the problem to the introspective method, account, probably, for the pre-dominance of inductive method used by numerous investigators of this field. The difficulty encountered with this method is in the enormously complex experiences which cannot easily be traced to the original stimulus; and yet a knowledge of the original stimulus is necessary if the analysis is to be complete. In this respect the deductive procedure may be better. This furnishes us with a comprehensive basis of general experience, of which the experience derived from music is but one form, and thus supplies us with a broader source-material than would otherwise be possible. Therefore, types will be classified according to their general psychological level, rather than to their specific character. Obviously, such an analysis will not always permit a classification into concrete types; but, on the other hand, it will embrace all types of experiences, and thereby avoid the necessity of adding new types to the list. If such an analysis is correct, it will have to include all the types already established, whether by investigation in the psychological laboratory or in everyday observation. And the availability for, and application of these data to the plan will then serve as a test of the adequacy of the analysis.

Many classifications of how persons differ in their responses to a certain stimulus or situation have been made. Many more are possible. Each classification has its advantages and its disadvantages, depending upon the particular point of view adopted. Some general classifications into two types are : objective-subjective ; knowing-feeling ; intellectual-emotional ; physiological-psychological ; analytic-synthetic ; reasoning-intuitive ; trained-untrained. Other classifications are : enumerative, observational, emotional, erudite ; or sensational, physiological, emotional, objective, character ; or analytic, motor, imaginative, emotional. Many of the classifications mentioned represent differences in terms only, for example, the knowing-feeling, and the intellectual-emotional division. In fact, this distinction between the knowing and the feeling is not only the most frequently found distinction in the classification of types made under control conditions, but represents also the most popular classification among musicians and laymen. The familiar sentence : " his technique is flawless, but his playing lacks feeling " is the typical expression of this distinction. But a classification into two such types is too general to serve the purposes of an adequate analysis. The physiological-psychological classification, generally speaking, represents about the same distinction, in popular parlance, as does the objective-subjective. In all these classifications, the subjective or feeling aspect is often intended to cover a vague, unanalyzable experience : the so-called intuitive response. But if we admit intuition, further analysis is useless. Moreover, it can be shown that what we call intuition is a very rapidly executed objective response, the separate stages of which we were conscious of when the response was originally being acquired. We shall, therefore, as far as possible, avoid these and similar difficulties by considering types of responses, not as separate entities, mutually exclusive, but as stages in a continuous general process.

In our responses to objective stimuli, fairly definite psychological processes are involved, such as sensation, perception, memory and imagination. Although, as a result of the integrative action of the nervous system, as well as of the continuity of experience, these processes are not sharply differentiated, yet they convey a sufficiently definite meaning to make them serviceable for our purpose. Since auditory experiences are one form of general experience, and since a musical response is one form of auditory experience, the psychological principles underlying our responses to music are the same as those which underlie human responses in general. The importance of conceiving the response to music as one form of response in general, inseparably bound up with the latter, cannot well be over-emphasized. This is our starting-point.

If response to music, then, be a form of general response and based upon the same principles as general response, a plan for types of response is given in the plan of general response accepted by general psychology. From this plan I shall select three processes : sensation, perception, and imagination as best adapted to an analysis of our problem. Again it is advisable to warn against a conception of these types as absolutely fixed and clearly differentiated entities. Human behaviour does not work that way. Nevertheless, the types mentioned have a sufficiently widespread application to class them as differentials.

All experience may be divided into two classes : auditory and non-auditory. Strictly speaking, a non-auditory experience cannot be said to be musical, but that it has a function in music, and a highly important one, will be indicated in a later chapter.[1] Whatever may be the psychological complex operating in our enjoyment of music, it is by no means limited to the field of audition for its sensory material. Many factors in the musical experience simply cannot be explained on auditory bases.

Each of the two general classes, auditory and non-auditory may next be divided into the three types mentioned : sensorial, perceptual, imaginal. Briefly described, the sensorial response is limited to the unsystematized and ungrouped sensory material ; the perceptual to the organized or grouped sensory material immediately present objectively to sense ; and the imaginal to the re-creation of this perceptive material through memory activity, or the creation of newly

[1] Chapter XIII.

elaborated and varied material through the action of so-called productive imagination.

AUDITORY-RESPONSE

Sensorial Type

The basis of the sensorial type of auditory response is the raw sensory material. Responses of the sensorial type are limited entirely to what is given in the auditory stimulus itself ; and this stimulus is restricted here to a single tone, or an unanalyzed chord. The characteristics of such a stimulus are, in audition: pitch, intensity, duration, and quality, and whatever sensorial factor we find, must be explained as a result of the effects of these characteristics.

The psychology of the sensorial-response type is characterized chiefly by the absence of higher units. Each stimulus is experienced as a separate unit ; it is unaffected by the preceding stimulus and is without effect upon the succeeding stimulus. The character of the stimulus is thus independent of its environment, and although a pure type of sensorial experience is only theoretically existant, yet this type is frequently linked with others, and hence contributes to the general experience. In fact, when the single stimulus occupies the focus of attention and there is but little fringe, the sensorial response actually determines the effect. A discord is unpleasant, because it is not associated with its successors, either in imagery or in perception, an association which readily modifies or alters the feeling-tone if the particular chord succession is a progression from greater to less complexity of tone-form.[1] For a similar reason, the pleasantness attached to many high tones through their pitch environment, is lost to the sensorial type of response, which knows no environment. In other words, the pleasantness-unpleasantness

[1] O. Ortmann, "The Sensorial Basis of Music Appreciation": *Comparative Psychology*, vol. ii, no. 3, June, 1922.

effects of the attributes of tone: pitch, intensity, duration, and quality that may be present, remain unmodified by the operation of any higher mental processes. The sensorial response is essentially physiological. Accordingly we should expect to find it in animals, in young children, and to a less degree, perhaps, in unsophisticated adults.

Concerning animals, reliable information is meagre. The common observation that dogs howl when certain tones are played or sung is one instance of physiological feeling-tone. Such tones if produced *forte* will result in a more vivid effect than if produced *piano*, and the original selection of a particular pitch depends, among other things, upon resonance properties of the animal's ear. The effect of resonance upon feeling-tone is a two-fold one. If the tone is weak, resonance re-enforces it, and raises it to a moderate dynamic degree, which can be shown to be a change from unpleasantness to pleasantness. If, on the other hand, the tone is moderately loud, resonance increases it to the loud extreme, which is a change from pleasantness to unpleasantness. The extent to which resonance increases the tonal unpleasantness can readily be demonstrated. If the closely cupped hand be placed around the external ear so as to act as a resonator, and the high tones of a piano be played rather loudly, a region of tone will be found at which the sensation becomes decidedly painful. This tonal selection, the *Eigentöne* of Helmholtz, although it introduces a modification in the more general distribution of feeling-tone already mentioned, remains none the less proof of the physiological pleasantness or unpleasantness of tonal sensation, apart from all association.

The relative pleasantness of the middle pitch, duration, and intensity series, when compared with the extremes, is shown in the responses of young children to tones.

In order to secure some experimental data of this distribution of feeling-tone, three series of tones were given, and the children's preferences noted. Three pitches C_2, C^1, and C^5 were selected and were played on a grand-piano in good condition. Middle C (c^1) was then given three times, once *fff*, once *mf*, and once *ppp*. Middle C was also sounded for fifteen seconds, three seconds, and about one-tenth of a second for duration differences. Seventy pupils of various ages were tested. They were asked which of the three stimuli of each series they liked best, which least. The order in which the stimuli were given was from low to high, from loud to soft, and from long to short. In order to check the influence of order on the judgment the order was varied. The results show a minimal effect of order on this type of judgment. The following tables show the distribution of feeling-tone as found in this test :—

	TABLE I. Pitch.				TABLE II. Intensity.				TABLE III. Duration.		
mf 3″	Most pleasant	Moderately pl.	Least pleasant	c^1	Most pleasant	Moderately pl.	Least pleasant	c^1	Most pleasant	Moderately pl.	Least pleasant
C_2	13	13	74	fff	1	5	94	15″	20	40	40
c^1	74	22	4	mf	74	25	1	3″	90	10	0
c^5	10	63	27	ppp	25	62	13	1/10″	10	40	50

(20 subjects only.)

(The numbers given show percentile distribution.)

In all the tables the marked preference for stimuli near the middle of each primary series is evident. Of the children tested, the older ones found it very difficult to make a distinction. Their responses, in many instances, were less spontaneous and less certain. In a particular group of fourteen pupils, ten showed the normal sensorial affective response, and four did not. These four were all over fourteen years old and have had several years of musical instruction, as a result of which their auditory associations are already developed. " I cannot say which I like best, I like them all " ; " It all depends upon what the tone is meant to represent," are some of the typical answers received. Many of these older children asked for repetitions, others remarked that they probably would not reply in the same way if the test were given them again. Whenever a preference for either extreme was shown by a younger child—a response which was met with but seldom—an explanation was demanded, and this brought to light that in each case associations were functioning. " I like low tones, always did ; they remind me of church bells, that's why." " I like the short tone, because it reminded me of a cute little elf giving a jump." Several children were asked why they disliked the very long tone, or why they liked it least. " It's tiresome " ; " it's monotonous " ; " I get tired listening to the same thing." For the very soft one : " Too hard to hear " ; " I could hardly hear it " ; " Didn't know if I really heard it." These remarks illustrate the elements of fatigue and strain associated respectively with great duration and minimal intensity. In giving such a test as this, it is necessary to use extremes of the series. A soft tone instead of a barely audible tone will naturally show a much greater percentage of preference, since the strain of attention is materially reduced. Thus a group of five pupils preferred the soft tone to the *mf* tone when the former was played quite softly and yet readily audibly, because " it is so nice and soft ". But this preference vanished as soon as a *ppp* tone was substituted.

The sensorial effect is more interestingly shown in responses to consonance and dissonance. In fact, neither the sophistication which normal adulthood of to-day necessarily brings with it, nor several years of musical training, which, as we shall see, leads away from the sensorial effect, is able to wipe out this typically fundamental response. Table IV represents the results obtained for twelve classes of persons. Isolated intervals, separated by sufficient pauses, were used as stimuli. They were played at a moderate intensity, in the middle pitch region, upon a well-tuned grand-piano, without the use of the pedal. Duration of each stimulus was about three seconds. The subjects responded in terms of marked pleasantness, moderate pleasantness, neutral affective-tone (if such exists), moderate unpleasantness and marked unpleasantness. The twelve classes represent selected groups in so far as all were music students ; they represent unselected groups in so far as they include persons ranging in age from seven to adulthood ; in musical training from 0 to 5 years ; and in musical talent from very superior to very inferior.

TABLE IV

Interval.	Marked Pleasant- ness.	Moderate Pleasant- ness.	Neutral Tone.	Moderate Un- pleasant.	Marked Un- pleasant.
	%	%	%	%	%
Octave	38	48	11	02	01–
Perf. 4th	14	43	25	14	04
Min. 6th	22	43	20	12	03
Maj. 7th	01	02	11	28	58
Maj. 3rd	43	47	07	02	01–
Min. 7th	05	24	28	33	10
Maj. 2nd	03	18	27	28	24
Maj. 6th	21	55	17	06	01
Min. 2nd	00	01	06	18	75
Aug. 4th	16	45	23	14	02
Perf. 5th	11	40	28	18	03
Min. 3rd	34	52	09	04	01

Weighting the marked pleasantness and marked unpleasantness effects 100 per cent, and arranging the intervals in the order pleasantness-unpleasantness, we get the following distribution : major third, octave, minor third, major sixth, minor sixth, augmented fourth, perfect fourth, perfect fifth, minor seventh, major second, major seventh, minor second. This is substantially in agreement with the investigations of other writers. In fact, it is this distribution of feeling-tone that gives rise to some rules of harmonic progression.

In spite of the fact that numerous sources of error creep into such a test, such as the characteristic diminuendo quality of the piano tone, the effects of after-images, the anticipatory judgment, memory response, and local conditions, the distribution of feeling-tone in Table IV is much too pronounced and too closely in agreement with the facts of physiology and physics, to be explained on other than tonal grounds. The constancy with which this distribution is met is shown in Table V, which contains the percentile distribution of the total judgments of each class, the various classes representing marked differences in subject material. These individual differences, however, fail to produce any marked deviation in feeling-tone from the distribution already found.

TABLE V

Class.	Pleasant.	Neutral.	Unpleasant.
	%	%	%
1	53	16	31
2	46	19	35
3	47	18	35
4	50	19	31
5	46	19	35
6	57	16	27
7	52	17	31
8	50	21	29
9	50	19	31
10	57	16	27
11	48	21	31
12	59	18	23
Average	51·3	18·3	30·5

(The Classes 1 to 12 are not arranged in this table in grades of any kind.)

The main conclusion to be drawn from these tables is that in the sensory material for audition there is a distribution of feeling-tone which is relatively constant, and in itself, may influence any response to tones, whether the latter be presented singly or in the complex forms of music. This affective characteristic of the tonal stimulus is, other things being equal, independent of the individual. It is present for all types of auditory effects, though it enters into them in various degrees. Genetically, it is the most fundamental type of response, since it is, at least to a larger degree than the types to be described later, more general, forming an essential part of many responses and some part of all responses.

In spite of this general physiological basis, however, the sensorial effect is not entirely independent of past experience. The affective character of the auditory stimulus changes for the individual, although the change is slow. This is a necessary result of the essentially physiological basis of this response. Varied effect, or its equivalent : organic adaptation, which is a fundamental characteristic of all animal behaviour, is responsible for this change. A stimulus, not harmful to the organism, becomes indifferent ; and with indifference it assumes a neutral affective-tone. Or, a complexity of tone-form at first necessitating organic strain for its adequate registration, may, through many repetitions and organic adaptation, involve less and less strain, at the same time increasing in pleasantness. Thus it is that chords, which at first are decidedly unpleasant, grow less unpleasant as they are heard again and again. (This change must not be confused with the change that they undergo when responded to as a part of their environment.) Several hundred repetitions, covering a period of one week, were necessary to change the originally slightly unpleasant feeling-tone of this combination

into a neutral tone for a seven-year-old child ; two months of practice on a piano composition containing this progression :—

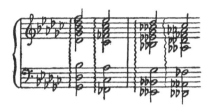

changed it from an unpleasant stimulus to a decidedly pleasant one for a seventeen-year-old pupil. Three years of acquaintance with modern harmony changed a teacher from an opponent to a warm admirer of modern harmony ; ten years did the same for another teacher ; five years for a third. The change in sensorial-effect witnessed in pupils as they continue their music study is an observation which most experienced teachers have made. One must be careful, however, in making a diagnosis, since in many instances the change may result less from altered sensorial response than from the substitution of a higher form of response for the sensorial form. A real change in sensorial effect is given by the historical development of music in which the development and application of harmony, apart from all questions of chord successions, form an unbroken progress from simple to complex ratio. Physiologically, this progress is equivalent to a transition from simple to complex sensation-form.

The sensorial response, then, is the typical response of young children, untrained adults, and untalented pupils. Of twelve adults, whose musical association was of a most limited kind, all found thirds and sixths

E

agreeable when compared to seconds or sevenths ; a distribution which remained also when chords, instead of separate intervals, were played.

Accordingly, we should expect to find sensorial pleasantness predominating markedly in popular music. A glance through this kind of musical literature will show this predominance. Thirds and sixths abound from " Feather your Nest ", " I'd love to Fall Asleep and Wake Up in My Mammy's Arms ", " Louisiana ", to the Italian Opera of Bellini and Donizetti (for example : the sextette from " Lucia "). Among other things, sensorial pleasantness of interval and chord structure is one determinant of the popularity of a composition. And probably the real cause for the popularity also of such pieces as Dvorak's " Humoresque ", the " Bacarolle " from the Tales of Hoffmann, " Holy Night," and " Juanita " is to be found in the emphasis placed upon thirds and sixths in these compositions. The affective tone of the unassociated musical stimulus is one source of musical enjoyment.

But, although the sensorial response is typical for the general untrained class, it is not entirely absent in the response of even the most specialized group, the pro-fessional-musican group. Kreisler or Thibaut need but draw a single down bow, Galli-Curci but sustain a single tone for sheer beauty of tone to become operative in the response of the musician. A vocal teacher, upon hearing a famous baritone sustain a single tone in a production of Rigoletto, exclaimed : " That tone alone is worth the price of admission." Again, when a sudden fortissimo breaks up any associative scheme which is functioning for the trained listener, the effect is essentially sensorial, forced in this instance by the intensity of the stimulus. And this is natural, since whenever a complex effect is present, its auditory basis is an objective stimulus which never really loses its priority claim upon the attention of the organism.

The predominant form of attention in the sensorial response is the non-voluntary or spontaneous form. Involuntary attention is present whenever extreme stimuli call it forth. Non-voluntary attention predominates because of the essentially pleasant nature of the stimulus ; for however unpleasant certain tonal stimuli may be, taken collectively, the pleasant outweigh the unpleasant. Normally there are more consonances than dissonances in the average composition ; more tones of medium pitch and intensity are used than tones of either extreme of the two series. In fact, when this preponderance of pleasantness is destroyed, music ceases to attract the sensorial type of listener. The essential urge for this type is physiological pleasantness, resulting from the natures of separate stimuli. When these cease to be pleasant, voluntary attention, this earliest and most fundamental form of attention, ceases to function.

It is not to be wondered at, then, why a child does not relish a Bach Fugue, or the average laymen a later work of Ravel. The attractiveness of these works lies elsewhere than in physiological pleasantness or its objective equivalent : physical moderation. Appreciation of such works demands the higher types of response which we have yet to consider. Sensorial response is characterized by a minimum amount of mental effort ; and the pleasure in this effect is within as easy reach of the moron as of the intellectually superior. This distinction explains why the average non-musical person finds pleasure in listening to music which the musician terms banal and commonplace. It explains the prevalence of popular music, partly that of *jazz* and the spontaneity of response of many musical audiences to compositions of a so-called lighter vein. In painting, we find the counterpart of sensorial response in preference for simple colour ; on the stage we find it in the cheap melodrama ; in literature, in the popular novel. The sensorial type of response is not to be deprecated as a device of the devil. Music can, in itself, be neither good nor bad. The sensorial response is a psychological necessity ; it forms the sole type of response of which man originally is capable. Training and education may lead away from it, but it remains the absolutely indispensable source upon which all later developments depend.

Perceptual Type

The perceptual response may be described as the interpretation of the sensorial effect. The sensorial effect is essentially concerned with qualities, which explains its marked affectiveness. In its pure form it contains little else than the pleasant-unpleasant distribution. The perceptual response, on the other hand, is concerned with auditory things : progression, sequence, motive, phrase, form, outline, contrast, ascent, descent, movement, and many others. Both types have a common basis in sense-organ stimulation, in which respect they are marked off rather definitely from the types yet to be considered. The basic difference between the perceptual and the sensorial responses is the presence in the former and the absence in the latter of relationships. The sensorial response represents a single impression upon consciousness. In the perceptual response, the effect of each separate stimulus is determined by its environment. What has preceded the present stimulus leaves its influence upon it. A tone now becomes a part of a melody, a chord becomes a part of a tonality, and a phrase becomes part of a form.

The psychological basis of the perceptual type of reaction is given in the psychology of higher-units. Consciousness never consists of one absolutely clear impression. Instead, it combines with one most clear impression many others of less degrees of clearness. These latter constitute the so-called fringe of consciousness. Reaction in higher units produces for consciousness the spatial and temporal series. The prime essential for a psychological series is an overlapping or at least a linking of one stimulus with the next. Stimulation separately produced physically, are grouped in consciousness into a psychological unit. The principles upon which the formation of higher units depends are the principles of the various types of association.

Accordingly, we speak of the span of consciousness. In the sense here used, this span is restricted to stimuli objectively present, and hence excludes the operation of memory proper and of imagination. The span is determined entirely by the objective stimulus, and may be described as a cortical after-image. It is the equivalent, in a way, of the specious present of James. Thus perception is used in its narrow psychological sense, and not in the wider popular sense in which it may be entirely independent of sense-organ stimulation. The requisites for the perceptual reaction, thus understood, are : a series of objective stimuli and synthesis of these into a single unit of consciousness. Stated in musical terms, this means that the reaction to an auditory stimulus is determined by preceding and succeeding auditory stimuli. A tone is reacted to as part of its environment, the E in the progression C–D–E is a different E than that in the progression C♯–D–E.

Evidence in support of the reality of the auditory-perceptual type of response falls into three classes : general psychological, musical-historical, and experimental. Since perception is a form of reaction in general, that is to say, since it functions in other sense departments, and since audition is but one form of sensory response, this in itself strongly suggests perceptual response to music. In fact, an adequate psychology of music will have to permit application of its principles to other sensory fields. The musical-historical evidence is found in the selectiveness shown by composers and in the treatises on harmony. Melody, harmony and rhythm, the three elements of artistic music are all perceptive terms. Melody can be present in consciousness only if the response to a first tone carries over into the response of a second tone. Harmony, in its artistic form, exists only if a preceding chord *leads into* a succeeding chord ; and rhythm exists only when the time distances between at least three pulses are given. This leads to an important conclusion : that any effect involving the attributes of melody, harmony, or rhythm, is basically a perceptual effect. Without perception there can be no melody, no harmony, no rhythm. The rule of melodic and harmonic succession, and of rhythmic diversity have been formulated as a result of the existence of perceptual reaction. If the chord progression G–H–I–J–K is good, and that of K–J–I–H–G is poor, musically, and if each chord separately is acceptable, then the order is the only reason for making the distinction. Order means series, and serial response, we saw, is perceptual response. The restrictions placed upon connexions of triads and other chords, the rules for sixth-chord successions, the distinction between the passing four-sixth chord and the cadential four-sixth chord, are entirely the result of our

responding to tones perceptually. The musical inadequacy
of any fixed system of figured bass is thus shown. A chord
has as many musical functions as it has environments ;
a tone as many as it has neighbouring tones. But as in
consciousness there is a difference in clearness in the
elements of the higher-unit, so, in audition, not all tones
or chords will have equal importance in the perceptual
response. Principality and subordination, or relativity,
is at the basis of all musical theory and practice, from
the psychology of Lipps, Weinmann, Bingham, and
Meyer, to the treatises of Goetschius, Robinson, Hull,
and Strube ; from the rhythm of Bolton, Squire,
Meumann, to that of Bücher, Hauptmann, and Riemann ;
from the harmony of Rameau, Helmholtz, and Stumpf,
to that of d'Indy, Debussy, and Scriabin. All these
theories and their application reflect the widespread
operation of perceptual response.

The experimental evidence for this type of response is
found in the recorded effects upon persons as well as in
their introspections. When tones are given on the piano
in non-tonality, that is to say, in an unfamiliar environment, and when these tones follow one another at the
rate of approximately one per second, the memory span,
or the number of tones that is held as a unity in consciousness varies from two, for very young and auditorially
weak persons, to six and seven for older or talented
persons. When a single tone is given and followed by
other tones in unfamiliar tonality at the rate of one per
second, with a pause of a second between, the period
through which it is judged *same as* or *different than* has
been found to vary from five seconds to twenty-one and
over, according to the memory span of the particular
person. The span for rhythmic patterns depends upon
the particular patterns used, the tempo, and the method

of presentation. When a quarter note has the duration
of one half-second, the span for a certain series of patterns
has been found to vary from

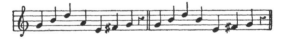

when the rhythms are given without accent.

The influence of environment upon a single stimulus
is illustrated when an attempt is made to secure a test
for harmonic memory span. The results of such a test
indicate, beyond any doubt, that the effect is not purely
harmonic, but contains, in many cases, a melodic dis-
crimination on which the judgment is based. Thus in a

chord group such as the following

the sequence is marked for a number of persons, by the

melody :

That such modes of response were used, was shown not
only by the collective distribution of the answers, but also
by individual replies of mature persons, who hummed the
melodic line when asked to hum what they had heard.
In comparing melodies such as

individuals frequently respond to the fifth tone, instead
of to the fourth tone as the changed tone. The size
of the interval between the fourth and the fifth tone in
the second example, marked in comparison to the remaining intervals of this melody, is the basis for judgment,
as is shown by the introspections obtained. " It was
separated more from the first four tones " ; " the melody
jumped at this point," are illustrations. Again, when

a series of melodies of the same length and pitch range
are given as stimuli, marked difference in the percentages
of correct memory span are found according to the
particular tone or tones changed. If the tones of the
melody were responded to separately, this could not
occur, since individual differences would function as
compensating errors in an unselected group. The actual
distribution found for ten melodies each of which consisted of five tones, played at the rate of one per second
in non-tonality was : ·19, ·58, ·60, ·68, ·63, ·03, ·54, ·74,
·10, ·77. The bases for these differences in melodic
perception as revealed by this test were : 1, Sameness
v. difference of pitch ; 2, Change in direction (ascent *v.*
descent) ; 3, First and last tones, highest and lowest
tones ; 4, Extent of change (quantity) ; 5, Subdivision
into tonality fragments (C–D as part of C major, F♯–G♯
as part of E major, or as 6 and 7 of A minor-melodic) ;

6, Pitch proximity, in which 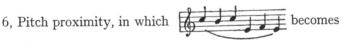 becomes

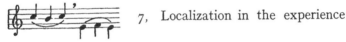 7, Localization in the experience

series (association with some familiar melodic fragment).

The introspections of persons in tests of musical response
are rich in perceptual types, since any element involving
melody or rhythm is perceptual in nature. The pre-
dominance of movement found in the introspections is a
reflexion of either rhythmic or melodic perception, which
forms the greater part of the usual auditory response.
In fact, every detailed introspective report contains
some element of perceptual response. A glance through
the literature is all that is needed to prove this. Sentences
such as : " I know I did it differently ; it all depends
upon what goes before and what comes after " ; " I do

not know whether it is the one chord which I am answering for, or the whole group " ; " I recognized the chord clearly before, but this time it comes in such a funny place that it sounds like a different chord " ; " I cannot hear the one chord without thinking of the others " ; " What a foolish question ! a chord never sounds twice exactly the same to me," are typical instances, picked at random from the introspection of pupils.

Attention in the Perceptual Response

Since perception is a conscious process demanding for its proper operation both analysis and synthesis, it is accompanied by active or voluntary attention. It means a response to the stimulus different from the nature of the stimulus itself. This added increment is the result of sustained concentration or mental work. Perception and active attention are so closely interwoven that we can properly substitute one word for the other in not a few instances. Consequently, the physiological con-comitants of active attention are also those of perception. " When I go to a concert," said an intelligent, normally talented pupil, " I don't want to think, I want to sit back and enjoy the music. I'll never be a musical highbrow." Since perception is the means of responding to higher-units, it involves a holding in consciousness of the sensation after the objective stimulus has vanished. And not a holding of one sensation only, but of several sensa-tions. This is essentially the mechanism of thought. It is true that the physiology of the perceptual response gives us a minimal group which is characterized by passive attention—just as the visual after-image is present without active attention—but this is only the lower extreme and plays but an insignificant part in the perceptual response. Moreover, perception is more often a deliberate process than a method of trial and error. It is a response through an environment which emphasizes one aspect at the expense of others. All this is essentially a product of active attention. The latter remains at the bottom of perceptual response. Nor does the transformation of fully developed percepts into habits invalidate this, for when we respond habitually, the content of consciousness is different from that accompanying perceptual response; and for our purposes here we may say that we have ceased to respond perceptually. This correlation of passive attention with the sensorial response and of active attention with the perceptual response is so marked that a change in the form of attention carries with it a change in the form of response. When frequent repetition of the same stimuli have made the original analysis and synthesis superfluous, our responses become essentially sensorial in type, in which a neural-complex functioning as a unity, takes the place of the reflex characterizing the sensorial response already described. And conversely, although perceptual response, and, through it, active attention, is essentially the response and attitude of the musically trained, the same type of attention is not always absent in the attitude of the layman. He, too, has at least a semblance of musical idiom. This may not exceed a few rhythmic patterns, chromatic harmonies, and melodic outlines, yet these suffice to give some perceptual basis. He has acquired these not by dint of actively attending to the auditory stimuli, but by countless repetitions of chance impressions : the piano, pianola, or phonograph of the neighbour ; the street-organ, the " movie " or theatre orchestra, for instance. For not a few such sounds furnish cases not only of a passive attention, but for many of us, of involuntary attention, in which the stimulus forces itself against our will upon consciousness. We do not find the layman employing active attention, but find him content instead to appreciate the stimulus sensorially. And since artistic music demands a perceptual process for an adequate appreciation, the layman is uninterested in classic music which he cannot "understand". It is not because the layman *could* not understand, but because the effort in active attention required to understand is greater than that employed by this type of subject. An inexperienced, normal adult, A., attended a song recital for a musical friend, B., and, when it was over, remarked that, with the exception of one or two minor things, she had found it without appeal. B. then played through the compositions and pointed out various phrases, whereupon A. asked : " Was all that in there ? " This potentiality for educability in perceptual response exists for every normal subject. But it demands a higher, more complex mental attitude for its development than the sensorial response. The sensorial response remains, without qualifications, the original path of least resistance.

Feeling-tone in the Perceptual Response

To the pleasure-pain distribution of the sensorial response, the perceptual process adds the excitement-repose distribution. The latter, in the last analysis is merely pleasure-pain in the service of higher mental operation. Excitement is either painful or pleasurable according to whether the goal, immediate or remote, is painful or pleasurable. A goal is always involved when there is movement ; and there is auditory movement whenever there is melody or rhythm, that is to say, wherever there is an auditory higher-unit. The feeling-tone in perceptual response is thus influenced by the attention factor. Mental work, like physical work, is essentially unpleasant. And, since active attention is the basis of perceptual response, this type, stripped of the influence mentioned, is fundamentally unpleasant. This is shown in the remark already quoted, in which thinking is opposed to enjoyment. It is shown further in the well-known dislike of music which one *cannot understand.* In native feeling-tone, then, as far as this is determined by the type of attention, the sensorial type is pleasant, and the perceptual is unpleasant.

But the unpleasantness of active attention is counter-balanced by two other elements : the pleasurableness resulting from the new aspects which perception yields, such as form, outline, movement, rise and fall, strain and relaxation ; and the greater ease of perceptual response which experience brings with it. The biological function of the response in higher-unit is to minimize the effort expended by the organism. That is to say, the formation of higher-units tends to lead to the forma-tion of reflexes. As we continue to respond to the same stimulus, our response tends to become more and more habitual, involving less and less effort, resulting in a change in the feeling-tone of the perceptual response. This is originally unpleasant, but through the operation of familiarity it may become pleasant. The pleasurableness of responses undoubtedly based upon perception, results, perhaps, less from the added elements which perception brings, than from the change in the type of response. For an experienced subject, a normal perceptual response involves no more work than a sensorial response does for an untrained subject. The feeling-tone is further complicated by the excitement-repose distribu-tion, which in turn is determined by elements of expecta-tion, satisfaction, surprise, agreement, and so on ; according to which excitement may assume either a pleasurable or a painful tone. A treatment of this aspect, too, should follow, rather than precede, the third response-type, the imaginal. It is mentioned here merely to complete the three elements underlying the feeling-tone in perceptual response : attention, experience, and excitement-repose.

Distribution of the Perceptual Response

We have limited perception to the response to an objective stimulus, allowing later for the play of past experience in the response to the objective stimulus. Accordingly, training which, in this sense, is not restricted to professional training or study, but is practically synonymous with past experience, determines the readiness with which the perceptual response takes place. This form of response, then, is typical for the musician, the normal student, and the talented layman who has had rich association, as listener, with tonal stimuli. The perceptual response is an index of the presence of musical talent. Variations in memory-span are shown not only in the experiments quoted, but also in the common observation of the ease with which certain persons reproduce extended phrases after a single presentation. A span remaining the upper limit for one person, accompanied by pronounced active attention, becomes practically as effortless as a sensorial-reaction for the person who has a much greater span. This explains the pleasure of the musician and the talented listener in a response which, for the untalented, involves an effort out of all proportion to the result. Perceptual response, in all but a very primitive form, is largely absent from the response forms of the untalented person. This type of response is pre-eminently that of the talented person. Between these extremes we have the moderate presence of perceptual response among normal subjects. A subject of normal musical ability can, through training, develop a not insignificant degree of perceptual power. For the perceptual process accompanies all life, and if we can learn at all, we can develop in perception. The importance of perceptual development in musical response is in the fact that it furnishes an answer to the much debated question as to whether or not training in music increases our enjoyment of the art. That it undoubtedly does increase this enjoyment is shown by the vastly superior store of stimuli which the perceptual process ultimately furnishes. When a musician responds to motives, phrases, sentences, movements, harmonic sequences, and what not, with the same ease that restricts the layman to a single tone or chord, or at most three or four tones or chords, the former experiences not only the pleasurableness of these elements themselves, but also that of a great variety of associations, to which they give rise. If the talented person had to *think about* these things as the untalented person does, the perceptua response would remain essentially unpleasant. It is because the perceptual response for the musican partakes of the characteristics of habits that the response involves a minimum of work. Hence when the layman is confronted with a fugue, the appreciation of which demands melodic and formal analysis (since the incidental harmonies made by the simultaneous presence of two or more melodies are the result of melodic structure, in which respect they are to be understood), the effect is unpleasant because his perceptive faculties are not equal to the task, and we get the pun : " A fugue is a composition in which one voice comes in after another, and one person goes out after another." Again, in progressions such as the following :

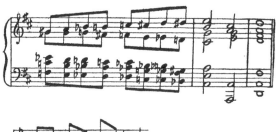

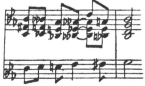

The vividness of each discord may cause an unpleasant effect so long as we respond to each chord separately. But to the person whose memory-span is equal to the entire progression, the movement into a final point of repose results in a different effect, all the chords becoming *leading-chords* into the final chord. Attention, being directed toward the latter, holds the others merely " in passing ", that is to say, they occupy positions more or less in the fringe of attention. The same psychological attitude holds if we respond to the melodic aspect of the example. Here melodic movement occupies the focus of attention, and the dissonances which the tone *chances* to make in passing along, stand in the fringe. These positions in the field of consciousness have different affective qualities.

The degree to which a subject responds to higher units is one of the most important elements, if not the most important element, in the auditory field of musical enjoyment. To-day, for the layman at least, the major and minor triads form the upper limits of consonance. They are also the basis of the music from Bach to Wagner. Tone combinations representing more complex ratios than these are, for the average person, unpleasant unless responded to in environment. The preponderance, therefore, of dissonances in modern music, explains the dislike of the layman for this type of music. Of course, when strangeness, novelty, and such things are responsible for a pleasurable effect, we are dealing with an association and not a purely auditory response. The associative response will be discussed later. Sensorially or physiologically, modern harmonies are unpleasant for the untrained listener ; which is but another way of saying that a perceptual process is necessary, or was necessary, at some time in the past experience of a listener, for a proper auditory appreciation of modern music. The same deduction holds for the appreciation of so-called classic music, which represents more complex structures than those of the popular music. Classic music (I use the term merely because of its wide application, psychologically it does not represent any type), demands a perceptual process when compared with the popular music, familiarity with which has enabled even the layman to respond essentially sensorially without sacrificing melodic and rhythmic impressions. The popular belief that the untrained listener enjoys music more than the trained listener is based upon the false assumption that the trained listener is constantly thinking about the music. This is not true. The training enables the listener to increase his store of sensorial response, and thus also to increase his sources of pleasure. The dislike of the musician for poor popular music is not the result of an ethically superior conception, but the result of the obvious nature of the progression, which no longer fills the demands which his improved powers of comprehension make. A musician is just as capable of enjoying a popular tune sensorially as is the layman.

F

Thousand-fold repetition of these simple stimuli has resulted in such complete adaptation that the original affective tone is all but lost.   Many musicians have had the experience of seeing the charm of their favourite composers during youth grow less and less as experience with tones continued.   This is but an instance of adaptation, and the effect thereof cannot be avoided

Imaginal Type

The imaginal type of response, as the name indicates, results from the play of imagery.   Perceptual response was essentially presentative, imaginal response is representative.   To the extent to which we allowed the functioning of past experience in perceptual response, we anticipated the imaginal type.   Since human experience is no more a series of separate units than the mind is a series of separate faculties, we have to deal with an unbroken process in which type differences are rather differences of degrees, or stages of development, than unconnected apartments and departments.   Nevertheless, the distinction between the perceptual and the imaginal types should not be lost sight of : the former is essentially physiological, based upon the presence of an objective stimulus ;   the latter is essentially psychological, based upon the presence of an auditory subjective stimulus.   To the extent that an objective stimulus is present in imaginal response, this reponse is perceptual in nature.

Concepts such as tonality, anticipated chordal resolutions, response to a melody *in harmony*, and the like, are results of an imaginal process in its reproductive form.   This is the most usual form of adult response to music ; and because the substance of this response exists largely in imagery, its operation is frequently overlooked. The extent to which it is operative is shown by the response to the usual forms of presentation of music—concert, recital, and so on, and by the data gathered in the psychological laboratory under controlled conditions. When, after a modern novelty, one musician exclaims : " Wonderful ! " and another equally talented musician : " Rotten ! " the difference cannot be sensorial, or, in this case, even perceptual. Instead, each listener brings to bear upon the objective stimulus an experience extremely rich in auditory and non-auditory associations, and the stimulus is responded to and interpreted in the light of this experience.

A test was given in which comparisons were made between phrases based upon our tonality system, and non-tonality phrases. Those tested were students of music, aged seven to adulthood; talent ranging from very superior to inferior. Two pairs of phrases were given, one for melody, one for harmony. Æsthetic preference was asked for. When the four phrases are combined the data showed that 92 per cent of the listeners preferred the tonality phrases, 8 per cent the non-tonality phrases. The distribution for the harmonic example was 90 per cent and 10 per cent ; and for the melodic examples 91 per cent and 9 per cent. This agreement indicates that melodies, although objectively the tonality need not be present, are heard no less *in tonality* than harmonies in which the tonality is objectively present. Hearing a phrase in tonality is nothing more than supplying an environment given by past experience ; an operation of reproductive imagination. If the æsthetic differences mentioned were sensorial in nature, we should expect to find marked differences between the melodic and the harmonic aspects, for physiologically the former is very simple compared to the latter. Sensorially, all progressions of single tones produced on the same instrument and in the same pitch region are essentially alike, for they all produce similar tone-forms in the ear. The pitch series is a continuous series, in which association of points rests solely upon pitch proximity. All periodicity, such as that of the octave, is harmonic in nature. Two non-tonality melodies, accordingly, should show approximately equal æsthetic distribution. For several classes of unselected persons the actual distribution for the two melodies given was 59 per cent and 41 per cent, which, when compared with the 90 per cent and 10 per cent distribution on a tonality basis, is a significant contrast. For the same reason a major triad was preferred 281 out of 289 times to a perfect fifth ; but only 129 out of 221 times to a minor triad. In the triad-fifth comparison, the triad was reported decidedly pleasant by numerous subjects ; in the major-minor comparison this response became largely one of moderate pleasantness.

When the following two chords were used as stimulus and the subjects required to note their preference and their like or dislike, 34 per cent reported the second chord of the example pleasing in sound.

When the following two chords were used as stimulus only 6 per cent reported the second chord pleasing in sound, though the chord is the same as in the first example. The second example is a progression from consonance to dissonance, and the latter, being interpreted in the light of the former, is unpleasantly tinged. In the first example this transition is absent.

In this case the response is to the absolute degree of dissonance, which, being moderate, is not very unpleasant. These illustrations, limited though they are, are yet sufficient to indicate the marked effect of environment upon the separate auditory stimuli. Moreover, environment need not be objectively present, but may be supplied by imagery as a result of training. Nor need the perceptual span be limited to two chords. It may and does extend much further, the actual extent varying with native capacity and with the training of the individual.

The effect of training, which, in the sense here used, is the equivalent of a reproductive-imaginal process, is seen by the following experiment, in which a consonance-dissonance test was given to a troup of trained musicians. The instructions called for a judgment as to whether or not the tone combinations (various intervals) were better or worse in consonance or harmony. With the instruction purposely limited to this description practically the entire group found it impossible to dissociate the stimulus from an imaged environment. " I hear that tone going up and the other down." " I hear a modulation into the dominant." " Tones of a minor second go together very nicely, they suggest a number of progressions to me." " Often I heard the tones leading to other tones, and when the next example was something else it did not fit." The tendency to respond to a stimulus *in environment* was so strong for this group of persons that only after repeated trials were judgments on the separate intervals secured, and then not without frequent reversions to type.

Distribution of the Imaginal Response

Since the neural basis for imaginaton is in the richness, retentiveness, and permeability of the pathways, and since the latter are determined by the perceptual process, we may expect to find the auditory imaginal response characteristic essentially of trained musicians and superiorly talented laymen who have had frequent association with auditory stimuli. If the perceptual response excluded the inferiorly talented, the imaginal response, which derives its material from perception, must likewise exclude this class of persons. The imaginal response selects from the broader perceptual basis those subjects capable of combining into new form their perceptual data, or at least capable of reinstating it in imagery. Thus it represents a more highly specialized group than the perceptives. This selectiveness is shown most clearly on the productive-imaginal side, where the composer stands as the most conspicuous example of the imaginal-response type. On the reproductive side the play of imagery is less clear to the casual observer, but here it operates for a much larger group of persons. Reproductive imagery is one of the chief elements in the determination of our appreciation of music.

The differences in degrees of perceptual response are paralleled by differences in imaginal response. When a musician is confronted with a composition written in an unfamiliar idiom, his response is, in a way, similar to that of the untrained person. For the higher-units of the musician cannot function efficiently here. One of two things results : either he attempts, with more or less success, to throw aside these acquired responses, or he attempts to force the new composition to fit them. If he does the first, then the musician becomes for all practical purposes an untrained listener, for with the elimination of his experience he becomes a layman and accordingly reacts essentially sensorially. He may enjoy the music, with the layman, on account of the changes in physiological sensation-form which necessarily accompany changes in pitch and fusional degree in the stimulus. He will not long remain on the sensorial plane, however, for the training which he has in perception will immediately begin to function. If, on the other hand, he adopts the second attitude, that of attempting to force the new substance into his acquired or habitual forms of response, the affective tone of his response will be determined largely by the extent to which the new idiom fits the old. This second attitude, as a matter of fact, is far more often met than the first, since it is impossible to exclude experience at will. But in the comparison and fitting involved in the second type of response, mental work, analysis, and syntheses take place. When the outcome of this work is a problem-solution, it is usually pleasantly tinged ; when the problem remains unsolved, it is unpleasantly tinged. This explains, to a great extent at least, the pleasure of the musician in a particular style of composition, whether it be the grace and charm of Mozart's, the rhythmic diversity of Schumann's, or the rugged chordal structure of Brahms' ; and it also explains, on the other hand, the displeasure found by many musicians in numerous new compositions. *The degree to which a musician enjoys an unfamiliar work, apart from its sensorial aspect, is determined by the degree to which this work can be brought into agreement with the idiom with which the musician is familiar ; that is to say, the degree to which it can be recognized.* The richer the past experience in variety of auditory data, the more numerous will be the points of contact—points where active attention begins to become passive—and the greater will be the enjoyment. To this extent the response of the musician to an unfamiliar stimulus differs from that of the layman; the former has a perceptual basis which in practice cannot be entirely excluded from new experience, while the latter, being without perceptual data, has no point of contact between the old and the new.

We are *disappointed* because, when all is said and done, the work did not meet our expectations. A musician after a performance particularly praised by the layman wrote : " I suppose most persons would find a genuine scream far more thrilling than a high C, but singing is art, not nature," words which expressed the sentiment of several other musicians. This is an instance in which the affective tone of the stimulus was determined by the attempt to bring it into agreement with a particular idiom. " I was much disappointed; he took such liberties with the composition; Chopin should never be played *that* way." Remarks such as these are too familiar to every concert-goer to need further elucidation. They all reflect the attitude which interprets the auditory-new in the light of the auditory-old, and they form an enormously large part of response types to music.

Since experience determines the play of productive imagery, the imaginal type represents a selected group. Since imagination, generally speaking, is a less common activity than perception in its extreme form, the imaginal response represents the most specialized group. But this class of experience is not limited to extreme mani-festations; it contains many degrees of productivity which shade back imperceptibly into the reproductive and the perceptive responses. In productiveness, it varies from the creativeness shown by changing a phrase such as this :

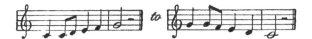

which represents a degree of productive imagination found in approximately 70 per cent of music students under test conditions, to the creativeness shown in an entire composition, limited to about 3 per cent of students. But quantity is not the only determinant.

A rhythm ♩ ♫♫ ♩ ♩ | ♫ ♫ ♩ changed to

♩ ♫♫ ♩ ♩ | ♩ ♩ ♩ represents an alteration very

frequently met, whereas its transformation into

♩ ♫♫ ♩ ♩ | ♩ ♩ ♩ ♩ is a much rarer change, and

occurred but once in several hundred tests. The lowest plane of productive-imaginal response, therefore, is broad, and corresponds to the lowest plan of perceptual responses. Both are relatively unselected. As we ascend the scale of imaginal response, we pass through various degrees of productivity, until we reach the highest level in the most individualistic compositions of the masters.

One further phase of imaginal response should be mentioned here, that is the extent to which the play of imagery remains in the auditory field. Since this involves comparison with imagery in non-auditory fields, an analysis of this transfer will be deferred until the non-auditory types are considered.[1] Two causes may be operative : the presence of an objective auditory stimulus may influence the play of imagery in the same sense department ; or the absolute amount of auditory data, when compared with that of other senses, may determine the extent of the transfer.

Auditory Sub-types

Variations in the degree to which we respond to a particular element of music : melody, harmony, or

---

[1] Chapter XIII.

rhythm, give rise to what may be called auditory sub-types. In the sensorial response, any one of the primary and secondary attributes may be the chief determinant of the response. Thus, pitch may be of greater effect than intensity, duration, or quality in a specific reaction ; or duration may be the chief stimulus. In the test describing the affective response to isolated tones, the hearers usually responded to the intensity differences more rapidly and with greater assurance than to the other two distributions. This supports the view that intensity is, in feeling-tone, the most marked of the primary attributes of tones. The maximal influence of an attribute determines the particular sub-type of response, for the three primary attributes are always present in every stimulus.

In perceptual responses, melody, harmony, and rhythm are added to the sub-types of sensorial responses, and we may speak of a melodic, harmonic, or rhythmic response in perception, according to the particular attribute that prevails for the time being. For subjects do not respond to the three elements equally. The facility with which they respond to any one may be greater or less than that with which they respond to the other two ; and, moreover, this preference may change for the same subject through the influence of attention or momentary mood. No subject represents a fixed type or sub-type. The response to a particular phase of the auditory stimulus alone determines the sub-type as melodic, harmonic, or rhythmic.

A similar classification holds also for the imaginal type. For the imagery, too, may be essentially melodic, harmonic, or rhythmic in content. Such variations in imagery are found in practically all detailed introspections on auditory response. In a test given for imagery, a selection well marked in rhythm yielded 446 titles, a selection less marked, 288 titles from the same group. Such differences are also found in the replies of the individual.

The lines of demarcation between the sub-types can best be adequately determined by experimental procedure, since it is impossible to separate any one of the three attributes, melody, harmony, and rhythm, from the other two. It is not that we respond to one element entirely, but that we respond to one element more than to the remaining two that determines the sub-type of response. Psychologically, the melodic, the harmonic, or the rhythmic responses do not represent marked differences, for they are all forms of perceptual response. The differences are found when we compare the sub-types of the sensorial with those of the perceptual or imaginal responses. That is to say, perception or imagination may be concerned with any one of the three elements of music more than with the remaining two, without changing the psychological level of the response.

CONCLUSIONS

1. Reaction to music is a form of reaction in general, and obeys the same laws. Definite types of reaction exist only so far as they exist in other sense-departments.

2. The relatively constant element in reaction-types to music is the psychological level at which they occur, for example: sensation, perception, imagination. The variable element is the individual, who changes in the mode of reaction with a change in the stimulus, and also with a change in attitude, and training.

3. Reaction to music is, psychologically, the result of a development rather than of a given state.

4. The determinant of reaction to music is native capacity plus experience and training. Training has a strong effect on reactions to music.

5. Training or experience increases our enjoyment of music. Any device tending to increase familiarity with artistic music is psychologically desirable.

SECTION II

THE SOURCES OF MUSICAL ENJOYMENT

Introductory Note.—The studies in the previous section pointed out types of listeners, their development and their æsthetic values. A further problem suggested by these studies is, given a person with a specific type of response to music, what are the factors, existing objectively in the music or subjectively in the mental and emotional equipment of the individual, that most readily call forth that typical response?

In most musical compositions one of the elements of musical structure, either the melodic, the rhythmic, or the harmonic, is predominant. The question is then specifically, does any one of these elements establish the typical musical response more frequently or more intensely than the others, or are all three elements equally effective? In other words, is any one of the elements a greater or a more frequent source of enjoyment than are the other two?

The papers in this section are concerned with phases of these problems. Dr. Gatewood treats them subjectively, her auditors being called upon to pay attention to the mental and emotional states resulting from hearing music of various types, while Professors Washburn and Dickinson's treatment is objective, their audiences being instructed to fix their attention on the music in order to determine specifically what element predominated in the particular composition, and its effect upon the listener.

As in the previous section, it is significant that the conclusions reached here by the two investigators are strikingly similar and supplementary.—EDITOR.

CHAPTER IV

AN EXPERIMENTAL STUDY OF THE NATURE OF MUSICAL
ENJOYMENT

Esther L. Gatewood

A MEASURE of the enjoyment derived from music, from one kind of music as compared with another kind, vocal music with instrumental and so forth, is important, but it is not sufficiently definite. Musical pleasure is too inclusive and may mean any one of several varieties of pleasure. One must discover not only *how much do you like it*? but, *how do you like it*?—*how does it affect you*? One may like the novel *Main Street* quite as well as *The Brass Check* or a series of articles by H. G. Wells, but in a very different way. Similarly, one may like Chopin's " Marche Funebre " quite as well as Debussy's " L'Apres-Midi " and yet feel a very different effect from each. The real problem is to analyze the sources and explain the nature of the different forms of musical enjoyment.

Four principal factors enter into the total which we call pleasure. The first factor is physical, and depends upon the forms of the music, described in terms of rhythm, melody, harmony, and timbre. A study of the direct effect of these elements is impossible as they do not occur alone, any more than do *pure sensations*. The other factors have, at an early age, become associated with this first.

The second factor is the associational and imaginal. If we call the first factor the *presented* content we may specify this second as the *represented* content.   Much of the music which we hear we have heard before, and because of this fact have associated with it a host of memories with pleasant or unpleasant colouring.   Even though we have not heard the given selection before, we may have heard all the elements of the selection, but in varying combinations.   The hearer may not recall the exact time or occasion on which he heard the selection before and yet he may have a group of images which are definitely referred to his own past.   Or he may have certain images the elements of which are from his own experience but which are defined as imagination, not being specific memories.

The third factor is the ideational.   The listener may, as the music progresses, be concerned with what we may call logical thought, either regarding the selection, its progressions, its structure, or with some other line of thought wholly unrelated perhaps to the music itself. The fourth factor is the emotional.   The term *emotion* is used throughout this paper very broadly and loosely to cover any affective experience.   It is with this problem that this study is chiefly concerned.   Simply put, the question merely becomes, what kind of feeling does the music give the hearer ?   What relation does each of the various feelings which the hearer experiences bear to his total musical pleasure ?

" I am Music.   Servant and master am I ; servant of those dead, and master of those living.   Through me spirits immortal speak the message that make the world weep, and laugh, and wonder, and worship."— Anon.

PROBLEM

The specific purpose of this study is to analyze the feelings reported by the hearer as experienced from listening passively to music and to determine the relation which the feelings and emotions aroused in the listener bear to his experience of pleasure or displeasure.

What kind of feeling or feelings does certain music give the hearer ? What relation does each of the various feelings which the hearer experiences bear to his total response to the music ? Can the individual's feelings be objectively estimated ?

Whether we consider musical pleasure as a unit towards which the various emotional effects are contributing causes, or whether we believe it to be a complex made up of the several emotional elements, the problem remains, what is the relation of the various emotional effects to musical pleasure ?

METHOD

One meets with an unusually difficult situation when undertaking experimental work with music. Carefully controlled conditions, which is the first essential in any experiment, are exceedingly hard to obtain. First of all, the material (the music) is of such a nature that one presentation is apt to be quite unlike another. For example, if a certain violin solo be chosen, one soon discovers that this performer does not play it like another, or that the same artist plays it differently on separate occasions. The use of phonograph music in large measure removes this difficulty. It does make possible a uniform rendition from time to time. The personal element, however, which is so strong a factor in some concert programmes, is necessarily lacking. The artist's smile, his gracious manner, and many other details which are active in the total effect from any legitimate concert are eliminated. This music itself is, however, standardized. All conclusions in this study are therefore based on music rendered by the phonograph. Certain general principles, I feel certain, are true of music in general, but one should remember that many exceptions may be explained on the basis of certain phases of an artist's personality, which are not reflected in the music itself.

Another difficulty is that of keeping any sort of control over, or measure of, the subjective element. Some observers are musically inclined, some apt to be temperamental. There is bound to be considerable variation in the mood with which the observer comes to different sittings. The experience of each individual varies and a certain amount of this experience carries over into the immediate situation. Some find difficulty in introspection, and are unable to describe or even to determine the effects of the music.

These difficulties have been controlled in the experiments on which this study is based by choosing three observers, all trained in introspection, by the constant conditions under which they worked and by the very large number of musical selections studied. Slight differences which might occur in the attitude or the physical or mental condition of the observer at various times are negligible when the results from nearly six hundred musical selections are used.

On a record sheet like the accompanying illustration, each listener recorded his judgments of each selection. These judgments were in every instance independent ones, as no discussion of the selection or its various qualities was allowed until after the data sheets were filled out.

	prevailing mood
	Title
	Catalogue Number
	familiar
	pleasant
	unpleasant
	interesting
	boring
	action
	memory
	imagination, fancy
	logical thought
	rest, quiet
	sadness
	joy
	love, tenderness
	longing
	amusement
	dignity, stateliness
	patriotism, stirring
	reverence, devotion
	disgust
	irritation
	rhythm
	melody
	harmony
	timbre
	technique of artist
	quality of record itself
	estimated wearing quality
	Remarks
	Name..................
	Date..............

The selections were played in sets of twenty each. Occasionally the number heard in a sitting was less than this number, but only in one or two instances was it more than twenty. This number is about as many as the observer can listen to, without the performance becoming perfunctory and arousing undue fatigue. The time allowed between selections for filling out the data sheets proved to constitute an adequate rest period.

Five hundred and eighty-nine selections were used in this study, chiefly those of a more standard character.

Explanation of Terms used in Data Sheet

Familiarity : 1. Low ; vague recognition ; awareness of having heard it somewhere before.

3. Medium low ; certain recognition, but not implying any familiarity with the parts of the selection, its title, or its production.

5. Medium ; certain recognition with correct association of title and melody ; recall of parts of melody, at least after beginning of selection.

7. Medium high ; recall of most of the selection upon presentation of the title, accompanied by definite associations and a warmth of familiarity.

9. High ; almost complete recollection of the music ; such a familiarity as would in many instances permit of reproduction of the melody and harmony by the observer.

Pleasant : In this column was recorded an estimate of the total pleasure derived from the selection. Zero represented a neutral condition, neither pleasant nor unpleasant. Pleasantness was recorded in terms of a scale from 1 to 9 as in " familiarity ", 1 being a small degree of pleasure, 5 average, and 9 the extreme of pleasure.

Unpleasant : This item represented the other end of the scale of pleasantness and was recorded in similar terms ranging from 1 to 9.

Interesting : This item represented the ability of the selection to hold the attention of the listener to the selection in and of itself, its structure, its uniqueness, its technical difficulty, and other such attributes.

Boring : Not merely uninteresting, but also forcing itself upon unwilling ears. It creates a desire on the part of the listener to remove the stimulus since he cannot ignore it.

Action : The extent to which the selection tended to arouse a tendency to movement, bodily movement, of some sort. This tendency varies from zero—none, and one—a slight inward tendency to rhythmic swaying, scarcely visible to the outsider, to nine—an almost uncontrollable tendency to act out the rhythm and movement of the selection.

Memory : The extent to which the selection aroused definite memory images. They need not necessarily be related to the musical selection itself, but they must have a personal ownership, a place in the personal history of the listener.

Imagination : The extent to which the selection aroused images unrelated to the personal history of the listener ; flights of fancy.

Logical thought : The extent to which the selection aided the logical thought of the listener, such as the solution of problems, the outlines of discussion, etc., or what is more often the case, the arousal of definite lines of thought about the systematic structure of the selection, its technique, its progressions, etc.

Rest : Quieting, restful, soothing, relaxing.

Sadness : Stimulating a feeling of sadness which may be pleasant or unpleasant.

Joy : Stimulating a feeling of happiness, light-heartedness.

Love : Arousing a feeling of tenderness or love, often through the words and meaning, but very often stimulated by the music itself, where there are no words expressed. (Includes also some meaning of the fitness of the music to express affection or love.)

Longing : Arousing feelings of longing for the home, friends, mother, or other loved ones ; creating a desire to experience over again some pleasurable experience of which the listener is reminded.

Amusement : Arousing fun, or a feeling of amusement, either from the content of the words, amusing situations, the incongruity of the music, or the grotesqueness of the whole, etc.

Dignity : Arousing a feeling of stateliness, serious solemnity, and an awareness of size, grandeur, dignity of movement.

Stirring : Arousing a feeling of either physical or emotional excitement, often accompanied by an impulse, to action for the purpose of releasing the emotional strain. Of this class, patriotism is one form.

Reverence : Arousing a feeling of devotion, worship ; the religious attitude.

Disgust : Arousing a disagreeable feeling of the inability of the artist to create the desired impression ; a feeling of the cheapness or sham of the production, particularly such as is noted when one attempts to be funny and fails utterly, becoming merely common.

Irritation : Disagreeable, annoying in timbre, technique, syncopated rhythm or other quality.

These eleven items are descriptive of the emotional effect experienced by the observer. For each selection, whatever emotions or feelings were experienced were scored and their respective amounts indicated in terms of the zero to nine scale, already described.

Rhythm, Melody, Harmony, Timbre : Each of those four musical elements were judged on the basis of the amount to which each contributed to the total pleasure. Not all were marked in each instance. Usually the one or two outstanding ones were scored in terms of degree of pleasure which they contributed.

Technique of the Artist : The quality of the artist's rendition, in a technical and mechanical way, and his success in artistic interpretation.

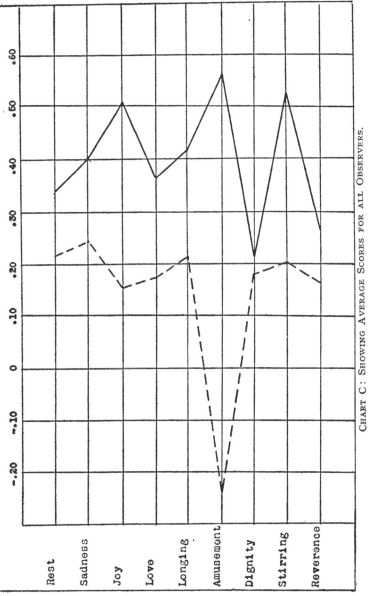

CHART C: SHOWING AVERAGE SCORES FOR ALL OBSERVERS.

—— Correlation of pleasantness with each emotional quality.
··· Contribution of each quality to pleasantness as a whole.

Quality of the Recording : The quality of the record disc itself, depending chiefly upon its smoothness and its intensity. The extent to which it distracts the attention of the hearer from the music itself is usually used as an index of its lack of quality.

Remarks : In this blank space were recorded any items or factors not accounted for under one of the headings provided, which influenced the judges' pleasure or estimate of the selection.

RELATION OF EMOTIONAL EFFECT AND MUSICAL PLEASURE

There are those who maintain that the pleasure which we experience from listening to music is a single unanalyzable psychosis, and that when we analyze the experience, all we do is to describe it in other terms. There are those, on the other hand, who describe musical pleasure as a compound, made up of various elemental feelings and emotions. Whichever may be the true nature of musical pleasure, the same problem remains. If it be a discreet, unanalyzable unit, the problem still remains of determining the relation which various other musical effects have to the psychosis which we call musical pleasure.

That there is an experience which we call feeling or emotion and that this experience often results from listening to music there can no longer be any doubt. Does this feeling, however, bear any relation to the enjoyment which we derive from listening to music ?

A study of the relationship of the degree of pleasantness to the *highest* emotional effect, regardless of the quality of the effect, shows a correlation of ·64, ·63, and ·54 respectively, for the three listeners.[1] This comparison

---

[1] Perfect correspondence between the effects as reported by two listeners would be shown, mathematically, by a correlation coefficient of 1·00. No correspondence whatever is expressed by the coefficient zero. A negative correspondence is sometimes found. The range of possible correlations is then from plus 1·00 to minus 1·00. A correlation of less than ·20, with the number of cases here studied, is rarely of any significance.

includes approximately five hundred selections for each observer. Not only are these figures significantly high, but the small range of variation between individuals lends reliability to the conclusion that some marked emotional effect accompanies marked musical enjoyment, to this extent. Other factors, the physical, imaginal, or ideational, or a combination of these may affect the total enjoyment from the music, but the emotional colour bears a fairly constant relation to musical pleasure.

A study of the relationship between all emotional effects for each selection and its score on musical pleasure reveals approximately the same. The correlations between the sum of all scores on emotional effect and the score on musical pleasure for each observer are ·64, ·59, and ·57 respectively.

Furthermore, the number of emotional qualities experienced varies with the extent of the enjoyment. Correlation of the number of emotional qualities scored with degree of pleasantness gives the following: ·67, ·40, and ·62, for the three observers' separate records. These figures would indicate that the selection which is more enjoyable arouses more different emotional effects than the music which is enjoyed but little.

The existence of a definite relationship between arousal of feelings and emotions and the arousal of a feeling of pleasure from music being established, there yet remains the problem of analyzing out the different emotional effects which the music stimulates and determining what relation, if any, exists between each emotional effect and the general effect of pleasantness or enjoyment. To what extent does the presence of a feeling of rest contribute to the feeling of musical pleasure or on the other hand in selections which give a feeling of rest is there a corresponding feeling of pleasantness?

Similarly, with sadness, with joy, and with each of the other emotional effects.

To ascertain this relationship we have taken all those musical selections which gave to the hearer a feeling of rest, for example, and have compared with their respective scores on rest, their scores on musical pleasure. All the scores on those selections which gave a feeling of sadness, were compared with the scores of these same selections on musical pleasure, and a similar comparison for each emotional group.

The amount of range between that quality which showed highest relationship to pleasantness and that which showed lowest is, for each observer, as follows :

Observer.	Highest.	Lowest.	Range.
1	·67 (sadness)	·29 (dignity)	·38
2	·63 (stirring)	·16 (dignity and sad)	·47
3	·55 (amuse)	·22 (dignity)	·33

It is significant that for each observer *dignity* ranks lowest in correlation with *pleasantness*, thus indicating that it is an element which may be present in selections well-liked or in those enjoyed but little. It is somewhat more vague and is less often experienced than many other feelings. It is evidently not so fundamental an effect, nor is it closely associated with pleasurable effect.

One must not think of these values as indicative of the height of musical pleasure from rest, from sadness, etc. They represent rather the extent to which musical pleasure parallels rest, sadness, etc., the extent to which when there is a strong feeling of sadness, there is a keen sense of enjoyment and when there is but little feeling of sadness there is only slight enjoyment.

Even with the wide individual variation, the averages

show a considerable amount of range. *Amusement* ranks highest (·55), *stirring* second, (·53) and *dignity* lowest (·22). The average values for each emotional quality are shown on the accompanying chart. The averages then show a range of ·34.

There is reason to suppose that a selection which is highly amusing would be greatly enjoyed ; and indeed this was found to be true in certain instances not included in this study. The difficulty here is that too few selections proved to be *very* amusing. Many people would find some of those same selections highly amusing and would enjoy them correspondingly. So far as our results indicate, the feeling of amusement plays only a small rôle in the total experience of musical enjoyment, but the extent to which musical enjoyment is related to the feeling of amusement when present is very marked.

If the correlations which the several qualities have with pleasantness are ranked in order for each individual, a correlation of these relative ranks show a considerable relationship despite the wide individual difference.

The relation between different observers' correlation coefficient are as follows :

Observers.	Correlation.
1 and 2	·34
2 and 3	·48
1 and 3	·57

If very great individual differences occurred we should find either negative correlations or no correlation at all. The positive values show that there are decided similarities between individuals in the *relative* amounts of pleasure derived from the selections which were reported to give the feelings of rest, of sadness, or other emotional effect.

SUMMARY

1. Other things being equal, those selections which show high emotional effect are most enjoyed.

2. Those selections which show several emotional effects are more enjoyable than those which show one or none, other things being equal.

3. Those selections the sum of whose emotional effects is great, show greater musical pleasure.

4. One cannot predict the kind of emotional quality from the score on pleasantness, for the simple reason that any emotional quality may be accompanied by marked musical pleasure. However, certain emotional effects are more often derived from highly enjoyed musical selections than are others, the relative correlation varying with individuals. For each of these observers, amusement is the least important factor in musical enjoyment.

5. There are marked individual differences in relative order, but the relationship of pleasure and emotional reaction for each of the nine emotional qualities is very evident. There is a decided similarity between individuals in the *relative* proportions of musical enjoyment associated with each emotional effect.

THE RELATION OF VARIOUS FEELINGS AND EMOTIONAL EFFECTS

A study of those selections which arouse more than one definite effect brings out certain facts concerning the character of the effects themselves. How is it that the same musical selection may arouse a feeling of rest and also a feeling of reverence, or what seems paradoxical, a feeling of sadness and a feeling of joy ? Can two discrete effects be experienced at the same time or are they aroused by different parts of the same selection ?

On the basis of the total number of appearances of each quality, *longing* occurs most rarely by itself. Whenever it appears— it is a concomitant of some other quality, most often *sadness*, and secondly, *love*.

TABLE SHOWING FREQUENCY WITH WHICH EACH QUALITY OCCURRED
WITH EACH OTHER QUALITY

	Rest	Sadness	Joy	Love	Longing	Amusement	Dignity	Stirring	Reverence
Rest		35		17	10		2		8
Sadness	35		4	18	25		6	4	7
Joy		4		3		8	1	23	1
Love	17	18	3		15			2	
Longing	10	25		15					1
Amusement			8					1	
Dignity	2	6	1						3
Stirring		4	23	2		1			6
Reverence	8	7	1		1		3	6	
Total	72	99	40	55	51	9	12	36	26

The right-hand diagonal half of the table duplicates the left-hand, but for the sake of clearness in computing later tables all figures are included.

Amusement and *joy* most frequently occur alone. In only twenty-four per cent of the total number of appearances is amusement reported as occurring with some other effect, and then only with *joy* and *stirring*. Of the total number of appearances of *joy*, thirty-two per cent are simultaneous with the appearance of other feelings or effects. Among these 32 per cent there is quite a variety—*joy* appearing with all other enumerated effects, excepting *rest* and *longing*.

It would seem evident, therefore, that a musical selection which is reported as initiating strongly the

TABLE SHOWING FREQUENCY WITH WHICH EACH QUALITY OCCURRED
WITH EACH OTHER QUALITY

(In terms of the total number of times the given quality occurred in the entire set of selections.)

Read down.

	Rest	Sadness	Joy	Love	Longing	Amusement	Dignity	Stirring	Reverence
Rest		26·5		20	17		10		22
Sadness	34		3·3	21	42		30	5·7	19
Joy		3		3·5		21	5	33	2·8
Love	17	13·5	2·5		25			2·9	
Longing	10	19		17·5					2·8
Amusement			6·5					1·4	
Dignity	2	4·5	·8						8·3
Stirring		3	18·6	2·3		2·6			16·6
Reverence									
						T			Y
Total	71	74·8	32·5	64·3	85·7	23·6	60	51·6	71·5

These figures mean that of the entire number of times rest was experienced (by all three) 34% of these times it was experienced together with sadness. In 71% of its total number of appearances it occurred together with some other effect.

feeling of *rest* will in most instances arouse also some other feeling, most often *sadness*, very often *love*, but seldom if ever *joy* or *amusement* or *stirring*. The feeling of *rest* is one without action to any marked degree, while the effects of *joy, amusement,* and *stirring* are fundamentally feelings involving some agitation, either physical, ideational, or emotional.

Stirring, which is experienced together with some other effect in the same proportion as it is experienced alone, appears to be in large measure the opposite of *rest*. It is never experienced from the same selection which arouses *rest*, and it does appear in many instances (33 per cent) together with *joy*. Also, those effects which are experienced most frequently with *rest*, namely, *sadness*, *love* and *longing*, rarely occur together with *stirring*.

The term *stirring* is an awkward one, for which, however, the writer has been unable to select a substitute. It is too inclusive a term, in that there are two well-defined forms of the feeling which is thus designated. The one is a physical feeling, involving an almost irresistible tendency to movement, the other is the feeling commonly designated by the expression " deeply moved " and is an emotional and ideational effect. Whatever bodily reaction is aroused, is of a very different character. The tendency to large external movement is lacking and only such smaller movements as the puckering of the brows, contraction or closing of the eyes, are evident. Changes in respiration and heart-beat occur, but these are not objectively evident.

The physically stirring selections arouse usually a desire to make large bodily movements, as for example to march, to dance or to mark off with the hands or feet, the rhythm of the music, although the body remains still. Such a feeling is often the sole effect reported by the hearer, or along with this effect may come the feeling of *joy*. In more than half of the instances in which the feeling *stirring* is noted with some other effect, this other effect is *joy*.

The emotionally stirring selections may arouse some other feelings, *reverence, sadness,* and *love* being the only ones reported, or it may occur alone. In this latter case, the cause of the feeling is unanalyzed, and the hearer is only aware of the emotional unrest which is aroused, without its taking a definite form. It is impossible to determine among those selections which aroused a feeling of stir alone just how many were physically stirring and how many were emotionally stirring, but it is certain that by far the larger proportion of them are physically stirring.

Joy, like *stirring*, represents an active effect as contrasted with rest. In only 32 per cent of the times that it is reported as occurring is it aroused together with some other effect, and 19 of this 32 per cent occur with *stirring*. In 68 per cent of the cases, *joy* is experienced alone. While *joy*, like *stirring*, is made up fundamentally of two factors, namely, the tendency to physical movement and an emotional feeling of *happiness, lightness,* and *joy*, it cannot be thus subdivided. The contributing cause or allied circumstance is often not felt, as is shown by the many instances in which *joy* occurs alone. Reflect how often one is happy without thinking particularly why he is happy, and even if he attempts to discover the reason, he is unable to do so.

Music creates a reaction not unlike that of poetry or drama. Save in the case of a very limited group of pyrotechnical selections, which have an ideational appeal, a considerable proportion of the pleasure derived from music is in terms of the feelings and emotions aroused. Certain reactions are opposed, and seldom if ever occur simultaneously. On the other hand, certain others rarely occur alone, for example, the feeling of *longing*.

In spite of the wide variability of individual differences

most selections producing any definite effect at all arouse the same in many hearers. This primary effect does not exclude the possibility of various other effects, varying with the individual, but it does show that there is a dominant feeling tone to such musical selections and oft-times more than one which is definite enough to affect all hearers more or less alike. These effects depend almost solely on the presented material.

In the selections which have one or more well-defined effects, there are less conspicuous elements which produce one effect on one, and a different effect on another hearer. Here the presented material is not adequate to arouse one definite effect and instead, the represented material from the hearer's previous experience and associations dominate the immediate experience. The affective tone is, in those instances, determined by the individual's own thought and mood, more than by music itself.

RELATION OF PRIME EMOTIONAL EFFECT TO NUMBER AND EXTENT OF OTHER FEELINGS AROUSED

A study was made of the relationship existing between the degree of uniformity of effect and, first, the number of emotional qualities experienced and second, relative quantitative scorings of these items.

On the basis of consistency, the selections fell into four groups. First, there were those which showed non-consistent effect. There was no agreement as to the emotion aroused in the various hearers. A second group contained those selections on which the reports from all hearers agreed on at least one emotional effect (sometimes more than one), but in which the average degree or quantity of this quality was scored below average (5). A third group contained those selections on which all the reports agreed, as in the second group, except that the degree was average. A fourth group contained those on which all reports agreed as to the emotional effect and in which the quantitative measure was more than average (7 or 9).

Among those selections which showed no consistent effect, fewer items are scored than in any other group, the average number scored being 2·65. Likewise, the average quantitative scoring is considerably less than that of any other of these groups. There is an increase with each group, both on number of qualities and on quantitative scoring, along with greater degree of consistency of effect.

The following table shows the increase in average number of emotional qualities experienced and the average quantitative estimates of such qualities, together with increase in consistency of judgment.

	No. of Cases.	Av. No. Qual.	Av. Sum Scores.	Av. Quantity per Quality.
No consistency . .	148	2·05	7·35	3·57
Consistency— Less than Average .	172	2·56	9·48	3·70
Consistency— Average. . .	66	2·67	11·17	4·18
Consistency— More than Average .	106	2·77	13·87	4·16

The meaning of these figures is briefly this : the quality on which there is the greatest amount of agreement is taken as the index of the consistency of the musical selection. If, for example, only one person scored the selection on *joy*, two on *love*, and three on *longing*, the figures on the last-named item, namely, *longing*, are used as the indicative ones. If all three scored several items, but the quantitative values for one are more than the others, the highest values are taken,

The score of consistency thus obtained is then compared with the number of items and the total quantitative scoring for all the items. It is found that those selections which have most pronounced effect have also other qualities in similar or less degree. Likewise the estimates of the emotional effects is greater in those selections on which all agree as to the outstanding effect.

It is often assumed that good music has one well-defined emotional effect and not a variety in small proportions of many qualitative effects. The contrary seems to be true, namely, that music which arouses many feelings is also more effective in its dominant or outstanding quality. The presence of many effects in lesser degree does not detract from the main emotional colouring.

An explanation probably lies in the fact that human emotions are not simple discrete experiences, but instead are a vast network of experiences, many subordinate feelings appearing as accompaniments to the emotion of which the person is most aware. The unstable character of our emotional experience permits rapid changes of entire content, and even more often a shifting in the relative intensity of the several emotional elements.

The composite feeling of which love is the most evident element, but which is not that alone, but is accompanied by joy, sadness, longing, or other feeling, may, in response to some stimulus, seemingly slight, so shift that joy becomes the dominant element, and love merely one of the subsidiaries; or so that sadness, longing, or even devotion, becomes the outstanding quality. The notable thing is, that when some given feeling is strong, it is not experienced alone, but has a large halo of other feelings which do not detract from the prime effect, but rather lend intensity to the feeling of which the owner is most aware. In order to arouse a strong feeling of any given

H

sort, it is not necessary to emphasize that one alone, or to remove stimuli to other sorts of feeling, but rather to arouse the desired feeling and also others not unrelated, which lend colour and emphasis to the prime feeling or emotion.

INDIVIDUAL DIFFERENCES

The wide variation between individuals, particularly in reaction to any complex stimulus, is so familiar that one is likely to question whether there are any general reactions common to many or all people. That music affects the hearer in a certain specific manner and that the effect is experienced, or at least may be experienced, by all hearers alike, is now fairly certain. However, from any stimulus so complex as a musical selection, a variety of effects and combinations of effects, is bound to result. The several hearers actually receive differently the same objective tones. The represented content of one individual's experience differs from that of every other individual. The emotional nature of one person differs from that of every other person.

If a group of people view at the same time a certain landscape, one of them may see only the ragged mountain peaks in the distance, and be held by a feeling of awe at their dignity and grandeur. Another may be interested in the sudden lights and shadows in the valley below, cast by great fleecy clouds gliding slowly by, and may experience a feeling of graceful rhythmic movement, with perhaps a feeling of joy. A third may be absorbed in the contemplation of a lone tree bent low by the persistent wind, and may experience a feeling of sadness and melancholy. Each of them may be aware of the various other objects, but he may be unconscious or only slightly conscious of their meaning or their affective tone.

Likewise each one of the group may be interested chiefly in the same feature of the landscape, the sudden rise of a blue heron from the river bank, and yet each be differently affected by the sight. The graceful movement may give to one a feeling of rest, to another a feeling of sadness, or the unusual experience may give to another a decided thrill of joy.

The same thing is true of the effects that result from listening to music. Not all people hear the same elements, nor do the same elements give exactly the same experience to each. I have made some mention of individual differences throughout this study in other connexions. Certain temperamental differences are evident between the several observers. These are perhaps best shown by means of a comparison of the total scores on each item of the data sheet. The musical training as well as the temperament of the three hearers varied. The observer with the least musical training excelled in emotional tendency. The following comparisons bring out these differences:

TOTAL SCORINGS ON " FAMILIARITY "

Observer.	Total.	Average.
1	1505	3·1
2	2143	4·2
3	2475	5·1

TOTAL SCORINGS ON " LOGICAL THOUGHT "

Observer.	Total.	Average.
1	48	2·5
2	34	2·7
3	1086	4·3

TOTAL SCORINGS ON " REVERENCE "

Observer.	Total.	Average.
1	384	5·3
2	232	4·7
3	340	3·5

Observer 3 was familiar with many more selections than was Observer 1, and to a more intimate degree. Further than that, her training had been such that many selections aroused some definite thought about the structure, the form, and other qualities of the music itself, and the technique with which it was rendered. On the other hand, in a purely emotional or associational reaction, such as the arousal of a feeling of reverence, Observer 1 shows higher scores. A complete comparison on the various items is shown in the accompanying table.

It is difficult to determine in some instances to what extent score values represent individual differences. It is quite possible that the score of "7" in one person's record may equal a score of "5" in another, so far as absolute intensity is concerned. In the correlations and comparisons of this study such a difference would have little, if any, effect, as all scores are compared with the individual's own scores on pleasantness, and the effect would be uniform throughout all of the items. In any event the deductions and conclusions would in no way be warped by this difference, even if it does exist. In comparison of one factor with another the same influence is present throughout, so that here again the effect is uniform and hence in no way changes the results.

The great amount of variation in the number of selections which each individual scored on each of the various items is interesting. More selections aroused a tendency to action in Observer 2, memories in Observer 1, and more selections aroused imagination in Observer 3. Only one emotional effect was experienced with greatest frequency by Observer 2, *longing*. Observer 1 experienced *rest*, *love*, and *stirring* more often than either

TABLE SHOWING TOTAL AND AVERAGE FREQUENCY OF EACH AFFECTIVE QUALITY

		Familiar.	Pleasant.	Interesting.	Action.	Memory.	Imagination.	Thought.	Rest.	Sadness.	Joy.	Love.	Longing.	Amusement.	Dignity.	Stirring.	Reverence.	Record Quality.	Wearing (Public).	Wearing (Individual).
Observer No. 1	Quantity Number Average	1505 503 3·1	2668 495 5·4	2290 497 4·6	577 183 3·	547 119 4·6	1860 408 4·7	48 19 2·5	1088 237 4·7	910 194 4·2	610 180 3·5	922 183 5·	433 80 5·2	155 57 3·1	494 107 4·7	698 163 4·3	384 70 5·3	2470 503 4·9	2451 503 4·8	2499 503 4·9
Observer No. 2	Quantity Number Average	2143 503 4·2	2813 503 5·6	2021 386 3·2	1006 222 4·4	377 98 3·9	1218 270 4·5	34 14 2·7	544 124 4·4	721 191 3·8	836 188 4·5	772 165 4·7	1088 215 4·9	166 54 3·5	327 75 4·3	604 152 4·5	232 48 4·7	2589 503 5·1	2984 503 5·9	2656 503 5·3
Observer No. 3	Quantity Number Average	2475 503 5·1	2549 492 5·3	1787 500 4·6	852 193 4·3	1298 282 4·7	1310 317 4·1	1086 255 4·3	1059 208 5·	1165 294 4·	1059 225 4·7	743 172 4·3	694 160 4·3	284 94 3·5	557 134 4·	458 108 4·3	340 96 3·6	2800 503 5·5	2406 503 4·9	1689 503 3·5

of the other observers. Observer 3 experienced each of the five feelings, *sadness, joy, amusement, dignity* and *reverence*, more often than did either of the others.

The individual differences shown in the extent to which each emotional quality correlates with musical enjoyment as a whole, has already been mentioned in another connexion. Observer 1 found *stirring* the largest element in musical enjoyment, and amusement the smallest. Observer 2 found *longing* the largest single factor and amusement the smallest. The relative order of the various emotional factors differs considerably for each individual, although correlation of the rank order for the various individuals shows a notable basic uniformity.

Similarly, in a comparison of the amount of pleasure correlated with each of the several emotional effects there is a difference in individuals, although there is a basic similarity, as shown by the correlation of the relative ranks of the several effects when compared with pleasantness. For Observer 1, *sadness* ranks highest with degree of pleasantness, and *dignity* lowest. For Observer 2 *longing* ranks highest, *dignity* and *sadness* lowest. For Observer 3, *amusement* ranks highest and *dignity* lowest. It should be borne in mind that these do not represent the qualities which give, or are accompanied by, the highest and lowest pleasure. They are rather the qualities which correlate highest and lowest with pleasure. Practically these may mean the same thing, although it is in no way a necessary deduction. Observer 2 was asked to name the qualities which he thought gave the most pleasure. He named joy, stirring, and longing, which three actually showed the highest correlation with the exception of amusement in his recorded analysis of the six hundred selections.

The importance of individual differences is shown in

the comparison of the choice selections of each individual. Each one scored approximately the same number of selections as giving a high degree of pleasure (7 or 9). The actual figures are :

Observer.	Choice selections.
1	239
2	250
3	236

Only ninety-four of these were scored 7 or 9 by each of the three. The remainder in each case represents the number of selections which only one or two observers greatly enjoyed. A considerable portion of this difference is accounted for in the terms of the represented material of each individual. In a song, for instance, the words may have peculiar meaning to one and not to another. A familiar melody may arouse very pleasant memories which contribute largely to the enjoyment of the selection. Fondness for a certain voice or instrument may be responsible for other differences of choice, etc. There are many details which enter into the total situation which we designate " listening to a musical selection " which tend to make the experience very different for various individuals.

However, individual variation is not greater in listening to music than in any other experiences. The individual likenesses exceed the individual differences. The use of music in all sorts of diverse situations by all kinds of people testifies to the great similarity of interest and pleasure derived from music.

CHAPTER V

AN EXPERIMENTAL STUDY OF THE NATURE OF MUSICAL
ENJOYMENT (*continued*)

ESTHER L. GATEWOOD

IN the preceding study we have pointed out that all musical enjoyment is derived from one of four sources : (1) physical, in terms of movement, felt to be either in the observer himself or in the music ; (2) a simple feeling of satisfaction not otherwise defined, usually dependent upon a quietly moving melody ; (3) associational, which includes emotions and memories ; and (4) ideational, which includes interest in, or analysis of, the composition, its interpretation or technique. The purpose of this study is to compare the four elements, rhythm, melody, harmony, and timbre, whether of voice or instrument, with these fundamental sources of musical enjoyment, and both of these with the reported effects of the music on the listener. The music material consisted of phonograph recordings of the following ten selections, used in the order given below :

Tears—Fox Trot . .	Tuxedo Dance Orchestra.
Scherzo-Tarantelle . .	Spalding, violin.
Volga Boat Song . .	Russian Balalaika Orchestra.
Shepherd's Dance . .	German, American Symphony Orchestra.
The Black Man . .	Sousa, Edison Concert Band.
A Dream . . .	Bartlett, Conturier, cornet.
2nd Hungarian Rhapsody	Liszt, Rachminanoff, piano.
To a Wild Rose . .	McDowell-Zoellner, String Quartet.
Volunteer's March . .	Sousa, N.Y. Micit. BO.
Ballet Music . . .	Orpheus, Gluck-Riess, Spalding, violin.

The outstanding features of the ten selections used, on the basis of plurality score, are as follows :

1.	Tears—Fox Trot .	.	Rhythm.
2.	Scherzo-Tarantelle	.	Timbre.
3.	Volga Boat Song .	.	Melody.
4.	Shepherd's Dance .	.	Melody (rhythm).
5.	The Black Man	.	Rhythm.
6.	A Dream .	.	Timbre.
7.	2nd Hungarian Rhapsody		Rhythm.
8.	To a Wild Rose .	.	Melody (harmony).
9.	Volunteer's March .	.	Rhythm.
10.	Ballet Music .	.	Melody (Timbre).

(Parentheses indicate close second.)

About thirty-five young women of the Lake Camp took part in this study as observers. They gathered together voluntarily for the evening's entertainment and most serious interest was evident throughout the experiment. Data sheets like the accompanying illustration were distributed. The observers were instructed to listen naturally to each selection, then at the close of each number to mark on the data sheet their reports by checking in the appropriate column. The material on the data sheets is divided into four groups and each listener was asked to check only one term of each of the first two groups, whichever term represented the pronounced characteristic. In the third group as many terms could be scored as were significant. The same was true of the fourth group, although it was not compulsory, nor even possible that any term of this last group be used for each selection.

PRINTED INSTRUCTIONS GIVEN TO EACH LISTENER

Listen carefully to each selection. Do not talk to your neighbour while the music is going on or at the close of the selections. Pay no attention to what your neighbour thinks about a selection. He may feel just as you do or he may feel different. The results on your paper must show exactly your own judgment.

Check one item in each group. Check that item which you notice most or which most appeals to you. For example, if when you listen to the first selection, the rhythm is the thing you notice most, put a check mark opposite rhythm, in the first column. If both the rhythm and the melody are marked, put an " A " opposite the *most* prominent one and " B " opposite the other. Do the same in each group.

DATA SHEET

Which do you notice most ?						
Rhythm	.	....	....	....	....	....
Melody	.	....	....	....	....	....
Harmony	.	....	....	....	....	....
Timbre or instrument quality	.	....	....	....	....	....

Why do you like this selection ?						
Feeling of movement in { you	.	....	....	....	....	....
{ music	.	....	....	....	....	....
Simple satisfaction and enjoyment.		....	....	....	....	....
(Cannot describe in any other way.)						
Images aroused (imagination) .		....	....	....	....	....
Associations aroused (memories) .		....	....	....	....	....
{ composition .	.	....	....	....	....	....
Interest in { interpretation .	.	....	....	....	....	....
{ technique of artist .		....	....	....	....	....

Did it make you feel :—						
Sad	.	....	....	....	....	....
Serious . . .	.	....	....	....	....	....
Like dancing . .	.	....	....	....	....	....
Stirred, excited . .	.	....	....	....	....	....
Devotional . .	.	....	....	....	....	....
Gay, happy . .	.	....	....	....	....	....
Rested . . .	.	....	....	....	....	....
Amused . . .	.	....	....	....	....	....
Sentimental . .	.	....	....	....	....	....
Longing . . .	.	....	....	....	....	....
Patriotic . . .	.	....	....	....	....	....
Irritated . . .	.	....	....	....	....	....

TABLE SHOWING RELATIVE PROMINENCE OF THE FOUR QUALITIES, RHYTHM, MELODY, HARMONY, AND TIMBRE IN EACH SELECTION

Selection.	Rhythm.	Melody.	Harmony.	Timbre.	
Tears—Fox Trot . . .	24*	3	—	2	
Scherzo-Tarantelle . .	4	6	2	19*	
Volga Boat Song . . .	5	11*	4	9	
Shepherd's Dance . . .	16	17*	1	1	
The Black Man . . .	21*	10	3	3	
A Dream	10	8	1	22*	
Second Hungarian Rhapsody .	14*	6	5	8	
To a Wild Rose . . .	1	20*	16	5	
Volunteer's March . .	30*	6	—	5	
Ballet Music . . .	2	19*	9	14	

* Indicates leading quality.

What relation does the dominance of certain elements bear to the nature of the effect experienced by the listener ?   Four selections have as the dominant quality, rhythm.   The emotions reported by most of the observers for each of these selections are as follows :

1.	Tears—Fox Trot . .	Happy.
5.	The Black Man . .	Happy.
7.	2nd Hungarian Rhapsody	Excited, stirring.
9.	Volunteer's March . .	Excited, stirring.
4.	Shepherd's Dance . .	Happy.

Selection four is classed dominant on melody by only one score.   The entire scoring was divided between rhythm, and melody.   The emotional effect reported by the greatest number of listeners for each of these is as follows :

3.	Volga Boat Song . .	Excited, stirred.
4.	Shepherd's Dance . .	Happy.
8.	To a Wild Rose . .	Serious, rested.
10.	Ballet Music . . .	Rested, serious.

Selections three and four show a very small plurality.

Two selections have as their most dominant element, timbre or instrument quality.   The emotional effects reported for these two selections are :

2.	Scherzo-Tarantelle .	Rested.
6.	A Dream . . .	Serious.

A more significant study is an analysis of the individual relationships between the rhythm and emotional effect, harmony, and emotional effect, etc.   With what effect is each element most often combined by the hearer ? Out of eighty-seven recordings of rhythm, it is combined thirty-five times with *happy* and thirty-three times with *excited, stirred,* a kindred feeling.   Complete details of the combination of rhythm with various effects is given in the following table :

TABLE I : RELATION OF RHYTHM TO INDIVIDUAL EFFECTS

	Tears Fox Trot.	Scherzo-Tarantelle.	Volga Boat Song.	Shepherd's Dance.	The Black Man.	A Dream.	2nd Hungarian Rhapsody.	To a Wild Rose.	Volunteer's March.	Ballet Music.	Total.
Sad	—	—	—	—	—	—	—	—	—	—	—
Serious . . .	—	1	2	—	—	—	—	—	—	—	3
Devotional . .	—	—	—	—	—	—	—	—	—	—	—
Rested . . .	—	—	—	3	—	—	—	1	—	—	4
Amused . . .	1	1	—	1	3	—	4	—	—	—	10
Sentimental . .	—	—	—	—	2	—	—	—	—	—	2
Happy . . .	14	—	1	7	6	—	—	—	7	—	35
Excited, Stirred . .	2	—	2	—	4	—	6	—	18	1	33

Total 87.

Harmony, which did not appear as the dominant factor in any selection of the group is but rarely scored. When it does occur, however, it appears with greatest frequency with *rested* and *serious* effects.

TABLE II : RELATION OF HARMONY TO INDIVIDUAL EFFECTS

	Tears Fox Trot.	Scherzo-Tarantelle.	Volga Boat Song.	Shepherd's Dance.	The Black Man.	A Dream.	2nd Hungarian Rhapsody.	To a Wild Rose.	Volunteer's March.	Ballet Music.	Total.
Sad	—	—	—	—	—	3	—	—	—	—	3
Serious . . .	—	—	—	—	—	4	—	—	—	3	7
Devotional . .	—	—	—	—	—	1	—	—	—	1	2
Rested . . .	—	2	1	1	—	—	—	—	—	5	9
Amused . . .	—	—	—	—	1	—	—	—	—	—	1
Sentimental . .	—	—	1	—	—	—	1	—	—	1	3
Happy . . .	—	—	—	—	1	—	1	—	—	—	2
Excited, Stirred . .	—	—	—	—	—	1	1	—	—	1	3

Total 30

Timbre, or the quality of the instrument, shows a marked relationship to certain effects more than to others. One must remember, in this connexion, that only a limited group of instruments was included, so that any results apply only to these instruments. The recordings in which timbre was most dominant are Scherzo-Tarantelle, a violin solo by Spalding ; and " A Dream ", a cornet solo. The most prominent effect of the former is *rested* and of the latter *serious*. Summing up all combinations of effect dependent on timbre in these selections *serious* and *rested* are the most prominent.

TABLE III : RELATION OF TIMBRE TO INDIVIDUAL EFFECTS

	Tears Fox Trot.	Scherzo-Tarantelle.	Volga Boat Song.	Shepherd's Dance.	The Black Man.	A Dream.	2nd Hungarian Rhapsody.	To a Wild Rose.	Volunteer's March.	Ballet Music.	Total.
Sad	—	—	1	—	—	4	—	1	—	1	7
Serious . . .	—	2	1	—	—	11	—	4	—	4	22
Devotional . .	—	1	—	—	—	1	—	—	—	—	2
Rested . . .	—	4	--	—	—	3	1	2	—	6	16
Amused . . .	—	1	3	3	—	—	4	—	—	1	12
Sentimental . .	—	1	1	—	—	3	1	1	—	—	7
Happy . . .	2	2	3	—	—	—	2	—	2	—	11
Excited, Stirred . .	—	1	1	—	—	—	3	1	2	1	9

Total 86

Our second problem is concerned with the relation of these same four musical elements to the basic sources of musical effect. Out of this problem two questions arise : (1) What is the dominant source of effect for each selection ? (2) Individually, what is the relation of the four fundamental musical qualities to the four fundamental sources of musical effect. The consistency of scores on fundamental sources of effect is more pronounced than in the scoring of any other group. For each selection on the fundamental basis or source of musical effect is as follows :

1. Tears—Fox Trot   .   .   Physical.
2. Scherzo-Tarantelle.   .   Ideational.
3. Volga Boat Song .   .   Associational.
4. Shepherd's Dance .   .   Simple satisfaction, associational.
5. The Black Man   .   .   Physical.
6. A Dream   .   .   .   Associational (satisfaction).
7. 2nd Hungarian Rhapsody   Ideational (physical).
8. To a Wild Rose   .   .   Associational.
9. Volunteer's March .   .   Physical.
10. Ballet Music .   .   .   Satisfaction.

In almost every instance there is relation between rhythm and physical effect. Three of the selections showing melody as the dominant element have associational influence. An analysis of individual records shows that by far the most basic source of effect correlated with rhythm is movement executed either by the observer or localized in the music.

TABLE IV : RELATION OF RHYTHM TO SOURCES OF MUSICAL EFFECT

	Tears Fox Trot.	Scherzo-Tarantelle.	Volga Boat Song.	Shepherd's Dance.	The Black Man.	A Dream.	2nd Hungarian Rhapsody.	To a Wild Rose.	Volunteer's March.	Ballet Music.	Total.
Feeling of movement in { you	11		1	2	4		2		13		33
Feeling of movement in { music	18	1	1	4	10		5		14		53
Satisfaction and Enjoyment . .	3	1	1	3	2				4		14
Imagination			1	5	2				1		9
Memories			1	2		1			3		7
Interest in { composition .					1		1	1		1	4
Interest in { interpretation .		1				1	3	1			6
Interest in { technique . .	1	3				4			1		9

Total 135

Several fundamental sources show about equal relationship to melody. Simple satisfaction and associational effect are equally prominent, with physical effect but slightly less so. The reason for the prominent relation of melody to the several sources of musical pleasure is the fact that melody rarely stands out quite so discreetly as some other elements. Usually rhythm is almost as dominant, in fact *there is no melody without it.*   There is, therefore, in such selections a combination of effect from two prominent sources. The selection called " To a Wild Rose ", which shows the highest score on melody, is characterized as having its effect on the associational basis. The " Ballet Music ", which shows the second highest score on melody, is characterized by most observers as giving a feeling of *satisfaction*.

TABLE V : RELATION OF MELODY TO SOURCES OF MUSICAL EFFECT

	Tears Fox Trot.	Scherzo-Tarantelle.	Volga Boat Song.	Shepherd's Dance.	The Black Man.	A Dream.	2nd Hungarian Rhapsody.	To a Wild Rose.	Volunteer's March.	Ballet Music.	Total.
Feeling of movement in { you	3		1		3		1	3	2		13
music			1	4	3	1	1	4	2	1	17
Satisfaction and Enjoyment	1	1	2	6	2	3		5	2	12	34
Imagination .			2	2	2		1	4	1	1	15
Memories .			3	2		2	1	7	2	2	19
Interest in { composition			1		4			1		2	8
interpretation .		2				1	1		1		5
technique .		5					1	1		3	10

Total   121

No selection of the group used in this experiment showed marked harmonic quality. From the individual records where harmony was especially noted those selections contribute a feeling of satisfaction together with a tendency to arouse associational effect, memories and imaginary pictures. Especially do such numbers arouse an interest in the composition as such (*ideational*) although none of these selections is particularly noted for its harmony.

The most prominent source of pleasure from Scherzo-Tarantelle, in which timbre is the outstanding feature, is the *ideational*, distributed between interest in the composition, the interpretation, and the technique of the artist, Spalding. The most dominant effect of

TABLE VI : RELATION OF HARMONY TO SOURCES OF MUSICAL EFFECT

	Tears Fox Trot.	Scherzo-Tarantelle.	Volga Boat Song.	Shepherd's Dance.	The Black Man.	A Dream.	2nd Hungarian Rhapsody.	To a Wild Rose.	Volunteer's March.	Ballet Music.	Total.
Feeling of movement in { you							1	1			2
{ music		2						2			4
Satisfaction and Enjoyment . .		1	1	1		3		7		4	17
Imagination		1	1			1		2		1	6
Memories						2		4		2	8
Interest in { composition . .								1		2	3
{ interpretation . .							1	1		2	4
{ technique . . .			1				2	1		2	6

Total 50

" A Dream " is *association*. This is a cornet solo of Bartlett's " Dream ". I am inclined to think that the effect is due in part to the melody and its unusual interpretation on the cornet. In this instance, timbre and melody show a combination where both factors contribute to the enjoyment of the listener in his feeling of quiet satisfaction. The selection is familiar to most people as a song, so that the recall of the words, as well as the past popularity of the selection, contribute to the arousal of memories and imaginative pictures.

TABLE VII : RELATION OF TIMBRE TO SOURCES OF MUSICAL EFFECT

	Tears Fox Trot.	Scherzo-Tarantelle.	Volga Boat Song.	Shepherd's Dance.	The Black Man.	A Dream.	2nd Hungarian Rhapsody.	To a Wild Rose.	Volunteer's March.	Ballet Music.	Total.
Feeling of movement in { you	2							1	1		4
{ music		1	1			1	3	1	1		8
Satisfaction and enjoyment . .	1	3	2	1	1	9		4	1	7	29
Imagination		1				3	1	2	1		8
Memories		1		3	1	4		2		1	12
Interest in { composition . .		3	1				1			1	6
{ interpretation . .		3	1			2			1	2	9
{ technique . . .		9					2		1	2	14

Total 90

What relation is there between the various feelings experienced by listeners and the fundamental sources of musical effect ? Are certain feelings dependent upon physical reaction, others upon ideational appeal, etc ? Specifically, is the feeling of movement accompanied by a feeling of happiness or a feeling of sadness ? Is the arousal of memories and associations by music accompanied by a feeling of excitement or by a feeling of rest ? A comparison of the fundamental sources of enjoyment recorded for each selection and the most pronounced personal effect or feeling shows the following:

Selection.	Fundamental Source.	Personal Feeling.
1	Movement . . .	Happy.
2	Ideational . . .	Rested.
3	Associational . .	Excited.
4	Satisfaction (associational)	Happy (Rested).
5	Movement . . .	Happy (Excited).
6	Associational . .	Serious.
7	Ideational . . .	Amused.
8	Associational . .	Serious (Rested).
9	Movement . . .	Excited (Happy).
10	Satisfaction . . .	Rested (Serious).

The relation, which source of effect bears to each individual's report, is a more important factor, however, than any discussion of leading effects ; for, what we are ultimately interested in, in any event, is the effect upon the individuals, as individuals. Certain feelings are evidently dependent on one factor more than upon another. The most conspicuous examples are *happy* and a feeling of excitement or *stir*. These are dependent without doubt on marked rhythm. Similarly the same two effects are noticeably correlated with the arousal of a perception of movement, whether it be referred to the person or to the music.

A feeling of seriousness is noticeably associated with outstanding quality of instrument, and, in addition, upon prominent melody, which is noted by the observer. Wherever an effect is correlated with the outstanding presence of timbre or instrument quality, special notice must always be taken of the instrument used. However, the instrument itself is some factor in the very prominence of timbre. In other words, the instrument quality is not especially conspicuous except with certain instruments.

The feeling of *rest* is particularly associated with dominance of melody and, secondarily, of timbre. This effect is particularly correlated with the experience of a simple satisfaction or enjoyment which may be something not yet explicable or may be a mere lack of definition. Observers often explain, however, that they cannot define the effect or the source of the effect otherwise than by the fact that they are merely satisfied, just as looking at a richly coloured velour may give a feeling of plain enjoyment.

We have not enough data on *sad* effects, but we are reasonably certain that there is no marked connexion between the feeling of sadness and marked rhythm. Rhythm is conspicuous by its absence in such numbers. Not enough material is available concerning sacred music to justify conclusions, except the absence of rhythm.

Concerning the feeling of amusement the results are not wholly conclusive, although these parallel those of all other observations, and show that decided rhythm and peculiar instrument quality are the two essentials for the arousal of this effect. " The Nightingale and the Frog," which is a duet between a piccolo and a bassoon, is a good illustration of this type of selection. One of the most certain sources of amusement lies in comic words, but our study of instrumental music excludes this factor.

Melody and timbre seem to be the two potent factors

in the arousal of the sentimental feeling. The relationships of all of these factors to each other are given in
the following tables :—

TABLE SHOWING CORRELATION OF EACH FEELING WITH THE FOUR ELEMENTAL
MUSICAL QUALITIES

	Rhythm.	Melody.	Harmony.	Timbre.
Sad		6	3	7
Serious	3	17	7	22
Devotional		1	2	2
Rested	4	19	9	16
Amused	10	3	1	12
Sentimental	2	8	3	7
Happy	35	21	2	11
Excited, Stirred	33	13	3	9

TABLE SHOWING CORRELATION OF EACH FEELING WITH THE FOUR FUNDAMENTAL SOURCES
OF EFFECT

	Physical.	Satisfy-ingness.	Associa-tional.	Ideational.
Sad	2	3	13	3
Serious	5	13	14	12
Devotional		5	2	4
Rested	4	23	11	17
Amused	8	3	6	5
Sentimental	4	2	6	2
Happy	35	12	12	8
Excited, Stirred	37	4	9	7

Conclusions :—

Conservative thinkers have long ridiculed the claims
of musicians and others that a melody itself may produce
a certain effect, that one selection may actually make
the listener sad and that another with a lilting air may
of itself produce a gay happy response. These same
people contend that a song without its words is devoid
of meaning.

The selections used in these experiments are all
instrumental and represent several types of instrumentation and musical selection. On the basis of a study of
the effect of these selections on thirty-five women,
the following deductions are made :—

Marked rhythm as an element in music is the chief
factor in arousing the feeling of happiness and the feeling
of excitement or stir.

Melody, as a musical element contributes chiefly to two effects, *serious* and *rest*. Prominence of melody is almost invariably accompanied by slow, inconspicuous rhythm. Melody of this type results in feeling of *quiet satisfaction* and *rest*.

Among the selections used harmonic effect did not stand out particularly prominently, so that no real conclusions on this point are justified. A study including a number of string quartets, such as those of Mozart or Haydn, might be more conclusive.

Timbre or instrument quality must, of course, be always limited by the relatively small number of selections used. Some instruments are better adapted to the interpretation of particular kinds of rhythms and melodies, so that the element of timbre rarely stands alone. However, that certain instruments have been selected for the orchestration and arrangement of music where the composer desired a given effect is well known. Proof of the ability of instruments to contribute to certain effects is shown in the large proportion of correlated scorings for *timbre* and *serious* and *rested*, on certain selections, particularly the violin solo and the cornet solo.

Various instruments will produce different effects. For example, the light tones of the flute produce a very different response in the hearer than do the tones of the cornet. The bass drum arouses a wholly different response. Likewise, combinations of instruments may produce a definite effect. For example, a duet between the piccolo and the bassoon is most likely to be amusing, but it is difficult to imagine a string quartet producing that effect. Serious contemplation and a feeling of *rest* are the usual effects produced.

The relation of the four musical elements to the fundamental sources of effect is not clearly defined in every instance. The addition of a great deal more data, on different types of instruments, and on selections where harmony is particularly prominent, is necessary to make deductions on these two factors reliable. On the basis of this study prominent harmonic effect is correlated with a feeling of sensual satisfaction and with ideational effect. The physical stimulation of the ear by beautiful combinations of tone produces a response not unlike that produced by a rich and beautiful melody. In addition, the combination of melodies and instruments arouses the ideational processes, particularly an analysis of the structure and composition of the music. The quality of the instruments which draws special attention to their timbre is such as to give a feeling of satisfaction and completion very like that which one experiences when looking at a bit of beautiful sky. Simple pleasure and enjoyment of the richness of the colour is experienced.

The appreciation of different instrument qualities is a genetic development. The grating sound from blowing through a fine tooth comb gives far more pleasure to the child of five than does listening to the magic flute, which he comes to prefer a few years later. The blatant notes of the cornet or the trombone are far more enjoyable to the youth of ten than are the tones of the violin. There is nothing wrong with the child's tastes, or his appreciation. The development of music among races shows a similar genetic development. It is probably a mistake to endeavour to *force* appreciation of the instruments past the logical order of genetic development.

Individuals differ in their choice of instrument

quality and in the amount of satisfaction which they experience from the same instruments. It is, however, significant that where timbre or instrument quality is particularly noted by the listener, a feeling of pleasure resulting from sense-satisfaction is also noted. The mere pleasurable stimulation of the auditory end organs may be the source of this effect. This same explanation applies to the otherwise undefined effect resulting from particularly prominent melody. The melody of those selections which show melodic prominence is usually simple, and the instrument quality, although not the most prominent element, is, nevertheless, a largely contributing factor, which appropriately combined with melody is the causative factor.

The direct relationship between rhythm and the arousal of a feeling of movement is ever present. The compelling force of some rhythms is more marked than others. Individuals differ, but whether the movement is referred to the listener's own person or is localized in the music, the effect is directly dependent on the rhythm of the music. It is probable that the physiological basis of melody may also be in terms of movement, but the periods are less marked, the direct connexion less definite, being in terms of slight rise and fall in dynamic balance.

Observers' reports show definite relation of the feelings experienced to the four fundamental sources of musical effect. *Happy* and *stirred* are usually related to feeling of physical movement. The feeling of movement may be of two sorts, (1) kinæsthetic, related to bodily movements ; and (2) in terms of imagery of the movement of the music itself.

Rest is that more or less neutral feeling which is most often correlated with source II, a feeling of simple satisfaction or enjoyment, and a general feeling of well-being.

Serious is about equally distributed between II satisfaction, III associational effects, and IV ideational effects. All three of these fundamental effects contribute to the serious mood. Sad, which is a more depressive feeling than serious, is most nearly related to associational influences, i.e. the arousal of either memories or new images. Many listeners, not trained observers, find difficulty in discriminating between memories and images not definitely related to their past. For practical purposes of analysis they form but one group. Both are represented material, aroused indirectly by the music. Some music may arouse the associational factor to a greater extent than other music ; some individuals are more susceptible than are others. The comparison made here, however, includes only those individuals who recorded associational effects and the feelings or moods correlated with these same represented effects. *Serious, sad,* and *sentimental* effects are all three related to the associational factors.

Not enough data on the arousal of *devotional* effects is available. One thing seems certain, namely that there is an absence of the feeling of movement (physical effect) when the devotional mood is experienced. No effect is dependent on a single musical element, just as no single musical element occurs alone. Each musical element is the contributing factor towards certain kinds of response. The corollary of this is that each effect experienced by the listener is dependent on a particular musical element or combinations of these elements. The music itself produces four kinds of responses, directly or indirectly co-ordinated with the prime elements of the music. These in turn are reflected in the personal effect which the listener experiences, and which are the only effects of which he is ordinarily aware. Rarely does the layman stop to analyze the source of the enjoyment which he receives from listening to music. He is satisfied with the fact that it makes him sad, and he either enjoys the feeling of sadness or else wishes for that music to cease and some other that will make him feel gay to take its place. He does not introspect carefully enough to know that it is largely the memories which the music aroused which made him feel sad.

In the previous study we have shown that individual differences in effect experienced are not nearly so great as has been commonly asserted. This study goes a step farther and shows that the personal effects are dependent on definite musical elements, and on the fundamental responses stimulated by these several musical elements in varying degrees. We are able thus far to define more closely the direct relationships of rhythm and melody to their effects, but that all four of these elements arouse definite physiological and psychological responses, which in turn are specifically interpreted in terms of the individual's immediate feeling or mood, is certain.

CHAPTER VI

THE SOURCES AND NATURE OF THE AFFECTIVE REACTION
TO INSTRUMENTAL MUSIC

MARGARET FLOY WASHBURN AND GEORGE L. DICKINSON

THE object of this study is, first, to note the comparative frequency with which the following musical elements : rhythm, melody, design, harmony, and tone colour, are mentioned as contributing to the enjoyment of instrumental music ; second, to observe the relation of pleasantness to the exciting and quieting effects of music, these effects being introspectively reported ; and third, to classify the emotions produced by instrumental music.

It was essential to the investigation that we should have a considerable number of listeners, and that they should observe the effects of a wide range of compositions. It is obviously hard to find a large group of persons who can devote so much time to a psychological problem. The difficulty was met by co-operating with one of the classes in the music department of the college, whose main aim was to become acquainted with the best music from Bach and Handel to the most recent composers. The number in the class varied from about forty to about fifty-five.

For the purpose of our investigation, each member of the class was supplied with slips of paper bearing the following printing :—

Number of composition.....................
(Ring the items you wish to indicate.)

Question 1	1	2	3	4	
Question 2	a	b	c	d	e
Question 3	a	b	c		
Question 4					
Question 5					

It was carefully explained to the members of the class at the outset, and they were reminded from time to time, that the meaning of these symbols was as follows :

Question 1 referred to the degree of pleasantness experienced by the observer from the composition. 1 meant indifference, 4 the highest degree of pleasantness. Some observers indicated intermediate grades by plus and minus signs.

Question 2 referred to the sources from which the pleasure was derived. The letter a referred to rhythm, b to melody, c to design, d to harmony, and e to tone colour.

Question 3 referred to exciting and quieting effects. The letter a indicated exciting effects, b quieting effects, c neutral effects.

Question 4 referred to any emotional effects not included under the heads of *pleasantness, excitement,* and *quieting.*

Thus, if a listener found a given composition extremely pleasant, she drew a circle around 4 of Question 1 ; if the pleasantness was felt as due especially to rhythm, melody, and tone colour, she ringed a, b and e of Question 2 ; if she found the music exciting, she ringed a of Question 3. Under Question 4 she wrote some such comment as *military, warlike,* or whatever descriptive term suited her more general affective response to the composition.

Question 5 referred to any imagery suggested by the

composition, but the data furnished here were not used in the present study.

The listeners were all young women. As a group they had had no special musical training, and consisted of individuals ranging from those distinctly not gifted musically to a few of considerable musical talent. The group thus represented an average audience of the cultural level obtaining among the students of a women's college. The observations lasted through the greater part of two semesters. Before the presentation of a composition to the class there was, except in rare cases, no explanatory comment on it. Afterwards, however, it was critically discussed as a part of the regular work of the class, which thus became increasingly sophisticated as time went on.

As a rule, piano music was reproduced by the Welte-Mignon piano player, orchestral music by the Aeolian Orchestrelle, and chamber music by the Victrola. For the sake of uniformity, our conclusions are based on instrumental music only, with the exception of the music of Handel, which was all from " The Messiah ". One hundred and eighty-two compositions constitute the list, distributed as follows :—

> Handel, eight compositions.
> Bach, thirty compositions.
> Haydn, seven compositions.
> Mozart, seven compositions.
> Beethoven, nineteen compositions.
> Couperin, Rameau, Scarlatti, one composition each.
> Schubert, two compositions.
> Schumann, twenty-five compositions (including the whole of Carnaval, each section of which was counted as a separate composition.)
> Chopin, thirteen compositions.
> Mendelssohn, five compositions.
> Weber, two compositions.
> Berlioz, one composition.
> Liszt, six compositions.
> Wagner, twenty compositions.

Brahms, eight compositions.
Franck, two compositions.
Tschaikowsky, three compositions.
Ippolitoff-Ivanoff, two compositions.
Dvorak, two compositions.
Paderewski, one composition.
Grieg, two compositions.
Elgar, one composition.
MacDowell, six compositions.
Debussy, four compositions.
R. Strauss, two compositions.

Results.

1. The Relative Prominence of Five Different Sources of Pleasure : namely, Rhythm, Melody, Design, Harmony, and Tone-colour.

Every case where a listener mentioned one of these sources of pleasure was counted as one point for that source. The totals were as follows :—

Rhythm.	Melody.	Design.	Harmony.	Tone-colour.
4151	5324	2814	2935	1558

For those composers who were most fully represented the totals were counted separately. These results were as follows :—

Composer.	Rhythm.	Melody.	Design.	Harmony.	Tone-colour.
Handel	119	144	137	65	235
Bach	446	736	727	352	179
Haydn	211	217	181	61	73
Mozart	135	203	153	59	76
Beethoven	492	522	338	332	190
Schumann	827	839	227	356	74
Chopin	382	466	220	234	114
Mendelssohn	134	202	78	116	49
Wagner	347	674	295	400	217
Liszt	133	173	59	157	92
Brahms	212	192	124	146	37
MacDowell	135	162	34	152	34
Debussy	94	100	22	124	42

The following inferences may be drawn :—

(1) Melody is in general the most noticeable source of pleasure, with rhythm next. Then follow in order harmony, design, and tone-colour. These results

probably do not indicate the relative amounts which these different sources actually contribute to pleasure, but their relative claim on attention. Thus harmony and tone-colour attract attention less than do melody and rhythm, but it is by no means certain that they contribute less to enjoyment.

(2) *Melody* was the most noticeable source of pleasure for all the composers except Handel, Brahms, and Debussy, for whom it stood second.

Rhythm was first in importance only for Brahms. It stood second for Haydn, Beethoven, Schumann, Chopin, and Mendelssohn ; third in importance for Bach, Mozart, Wagner, Liszt, MacDowell, and Debussy ; fourth in importance for Handel.

Design was first in importance for no composer. It stood second for Bach and Mozart ; third for Handel, Haydn and Beethoven ; fourth for Schumann, Chopin, Mendelssohn, Wagner, and Brahms. For MacDowell its rank was four and a half, and for Liszt and Debussy, five.

Harmony was first in importance for Debussy. It was second for Wagner ; third for Schumann, Chopin, Mendelssohn, Liszt, Brahms, and MacDowell ; fourth for Bach and Beethoven ; fifth for Handel, Haydn, and Mozart.

Tone-colour was first for Handel. This curious result is very probably due to the fact that Handel composi- tions are scarcely comparable to those of the other composers, because, with the exception of the " Pastoral Symphony " from " The Messiah ", they all involved choral singing. It is not improbable that vocal tone- colour attracts attention more than instrumental tone- colour does ; in any case the two are hardly comparable. Tone-colour was not even second or third in importance for the other composers : its rank was four for Haydn, Mozart, Liszt and Debussy ; four and a half for MacDowell, and five for Bach, Beethoven, Schumann, Mendelssohn, Chopin, Wagner and Brahms.

Since the number of compositions representing some of these composers was small, the above figures are not of great importance ; but in general they follow the recognized characteristics of the composers.

2. The Relation of Pleasantness to Exciting and Quieting Effects.

Compositions that are either markedly exciting or markedly quieting are more agreeable than compositions that are to the majority of listeners neither exciting nor quieting.

The average pleasantness of the thirty-two compositions found exciting by thirty-five or more observers was 3·22, A.D. ·23.

The average pleasantness of the 14 compositions found markedly quieting by thirty-five or more observers was 3·11, A.D. ·41.

The average pleasantness of compositions found neither exciting nor quieting by thirty or more observers was 2·42, A.D. ·119.

Thus marked pleasantness tends to involve a further effect that is either exciting or quieting.

3. The Dependence of Pleasantness on the Number of Sources of Pleasantness.

There is a tendency for the pleasantness to be greater, the greater the number of sources to which that pleasantness is referred.

Owing to the wide variety of the kinds of music used in the study, it seemed safer to calculate correlations separately for each of the composers most fully represented, than to find a single correlation coefficient for all the compositions used. The coefficients were found as follows:—The compositions of a composer were arranged in the order of their average pleasantness to the group of listeners. Then, for each composition, the numbers were added together that represented the number of times each of the five sources of pleasantness was mentioned. That is, suppose that for a given composition rhythm had been mentioned twenty-one times, melody thirty-five times, design eight times, harmony sixteen times, and tone-colour seven times. The sum of these numbers would evidently be greater, the more the observers had tended to mention more than one source of pleasantness in the case of this composition. The compositions of a given composer were arranged in the order of the size of these sums. By finding rank difference correlations between this array and the array representing average pleasantness, the relation between pleasantness and number of sources could be roughly made out.

The coefficients were as follows :—

> Bach, Plus ·47, P.E. ·09.
> Beethoven, Plus ·77, P.E. ·06.
> Schumann (Carnaval), Plus ·43, P.E. ·12.
> Chopin, Plus ·50, P.E. ·14.
> Wagner, Plus ·74, P.E. ·08.

4. The Emotions [1] Accompanying Music.

A very careful account was taken of every descriptive word used by a listener to indicate her general emotional reactions, under Question 4. The following classification includes all of these terms, omitting obvious synonyms. It is, we think, a very fair survey of all emotions which instrumental music suggests to ordinary listeners.

By far the most frequently mentioned emotional states

---

[1] The term emotions is here used very loosely to cover any sort of affective reaction except simple pleasantness-unpleasantness, excitement, or quieting.

were happiness, gaiety, calm, and sadness. These terms, or their equivalents, occur from twenty to two hundred times as often as any others.

Including these, the descriptive terms fall under the following heads :—

Terms referring to

I. Active emotional states.

    A. Pleasant.

        Diffuse activity : happiness, joy.

        Diffuse superficial activity : gaiety, frivolous, playful, humour, fun, teasing, mischief, whimsical, fantastic, teasing, flirting.

        Concentrated forward activity : exhilaration, stimulation, confidence, courage, certainty, triumph, force, power, purpose, martial, patriotic, encouraging, dignified, majestic.

    B. Unpleasant (slightly).

        Uneasiness, some conflict or inhibition present : hurry, unrest, searching, struggle, tumult, wrangling, confusion, bewilderment.

II. Passive emotional states.

    A. Pleasant.

        Calm, peace, soothing, reminiscence, contemplation, thoughtfulness, languor, sentimentality.

    B. Unpleasant (slightly).

        Sadness, melancholy.

        Slight element of activity present : something lacking : suspense, doubt, uncertainty, anxiety, longing, yearning, wistfulness, plaintiveness.

C. Involving slight fear : foreboding, weird, sombre, mysterious, eery, fear.

Since all of the comments which have thus been classified were accompanied by judgments ascribing some degree of pleasantness to the compositions that inspired them, it is clear that none of the unpleasant emotions indicated could have exceeded the mild unpleasantness which is compatible with æsthetic enjoyment.

All of the emotions occasioned by instrumental music belong to the type of affective reactions lacking a definite object ; thus they stand closer to moods than to true emotions. Love, for example, was thought by Darwin to be the source of musical expression, but love is not mentioned on our list. It requires a definite object, and the suggestions of instrumental music alone are too vague. Fear, on the other hand, may be felt with reference to an undefined object.

SUMMARY OF RESULTS

For young women college students, the source of pleasure most often mentioned in listening to reproductions of instrumental music is melody ; rhythm, harmony, design, and tone-colour follow in order.

For difference between composers, see page 124.

Compositions that are either markedly exciting or markedly quieting in their effects are pleasanter than those which are neutral. Thus extreme pleasantness involves a further effect that is either exciting or quieting.

There is a tendency for the pleasantness to be greater, the greater the number of sources to which it is referred.

The emotions accompanying instrumental music may be classed under the following heads : Active pleasant emotions, involving (*a*) diffuse activity, (*b*) diffuse

K

superficial activity, (c) concentrated forward activity ; active unpleasant emotions, involving some conflict or inhibition ; passive pleasant emotions ; passive unpleasant emotions (a) wholly passive, (b) with some element of activity ; emotions involving slight fear.

All unpleasant affective states are only mildly unpleasant. All emotions reported are without a definite object, and thus more properly termed moods.

SECTION III

THE MOOD EFFECTS OF MUSIC

Introductory Note.—Thus far we have learned the main types of attitudes towards music and the main sources of musical enjoyment. We are now ready to receive some light upon a third problem, namely, irrespective of the type of listener or of the musical element that predominates in a composition, or of the main source of enjoyment, what is the nature of the principal effect of music as a whole ?

The studies in this section are devoted to an investigation of this problem, and discuss it from many angles and points of view. In the first study, the nature of the main effect of music is pointed out. The second study is devoted to a discussion of the influence exerted by several subsidiary factors upon the main effect and the degree to which they condition its nature and intensity.

The studies are presented here as the joint products of Dr. Gatewood and Dr. Schoen, although conducted entirely independent of each other. The results reached by the two investigators were so markedly similar and supplementary that a united presentation seemed advisable.—EDITOR.

CHAPTER VII

THE MOOD EFFECTS OF MUSIC

MAX SCHOEN AND ESTHER L. GATEWOOD

Introduction

THE investigation reported in this paper was prompted by results obtained from a study of over 20,000 mood change charts on which that number of persons reported the effects produced upon their moods by a variety of 290 phonograph recordings of vocal and instrumental musical compositions. The tabulation of the data of these charts indicated in a most suggestive manner that, in general, a musical composition not only produces a change in the existing affective state of the listener, but that its effect upon the large majority of the members of an audience is uniform to a striking degree.

These results commanded attention, particularly in view of the fact that the data were collected from all over the United States from audiences gathered under various conditions of time and place, ranging from early morning until late evening, and from a police station to a church, and consisting of persons of varied musical training, experience, age and interests.

The validity of the above conclusion may well be challenged on the ground that the data on which it is based were obtained under conditions entirely out of keeping with established experimental procedure. The hearers were gathered for but a single session, and then in a haphazard manner, while the music material was selected at random, and the entire procedure handled by untrained persons. On the other hand, it is of utmost significance that even a most superficial examination of the data from the 20,000 charts, obtained even under these unfavourable conditions, points to the power of music over the moods and emotions. It was because of this fact, as well as in order to obtain more reliable data on the problem, that a further study along the same line was made.[1]

MOOD CHANGE CHART

Date of Test ....

1. Place ....
   (Home or Where)

2. Time (Mark x in square)
   Morning ☐   Afternoon ☐
   Evening ☐

3. Weather (Mark x in square)
   Dull ☐   Cold ☐
   Bright ☐   Warm ☐

4. What kind of music did you feel like hearing ? (Mark all words which describe such music with x)
   Tender ☐   Vivacious ☐
   Joyous ☐   Majestic ☐
   Solemn ☐   Soothing ☐
   Weird ☐   Exciting ☐
   Martial ☐   Dreamy ☐
   Gay ☐   Simple ☐
   Sad ☐

5. What was your mood immediately preceding test ?

   (Mark x in square)

   Serious or ☐   Worried or ☐
   Gay ☐   Care-free ☐

   Depressed or☐   Nervous or ☐
   Exhilarated ☐   Composed ☐

   Fatigued or ☐   Sad or ☐
   Unfatigued ☐   Joyful ☐
        Discouraged ☐
        or Optimistic ☐

6. As a result of the test, what were your most noticeable mood changes ? (Serious to gay, gay to serious, worried to care-free, nervous to composed, etc.)

   Mood Change   Selection causing such change
   ....to...........   ....
   ....to...........   ....
   ....to...........   ....

7. Please comment on manner in which mood changes occurred :
   ....
   ....
   ....
                        Signed ....

This further investigation dealt not only with the effects of music on moods but with many other questions on the same general problem. Thus, for practical purposes, we want to know not only whether a musical selection produces a mood change in the listener, but, what is of

[1] This part of the study is by Dr. Schoen.

greater significance, whether the induced mood is also enjoyed, and to what degree this enjoyment might depend upon such factors as the type of mood induced, familiarity of the listener with the selection, and his judgment of the quality of the selection. The problems upon which light was sought in this investigation, besides those relating to mood effects, are as follows :—

1. The effect of the induced mood upon the subsequent mood. Does an induced mood create a desire for its continuation ? To what extent does this depend on the degree of enjoyment derived from the selection and on the type of mood induced ?

2. What is the relation, if any, between the degree of enjoyment obtained from a selection and the judgment of its quality ?

3. Does a mood-change as such tend to produce enjoyment, provided the change is not due to such factors as poor rendition or dislike of the listener for that type of music, etc. ?

4. Does any one type or class of music induce a more uniform mood than other types or classes ?

5. Is there any tendency for any one type or class of music to be enjoyed more intensely than other types or classes ?

6. Is there any relation between familiarity and degree of enjoyment ?

7. Do selections familiar to the listener create a more uniform mood than unfamiliar ones ?

8. What is the effect, if any, of the listener's attitude towards his existing mood on the effect produced by the music ? For instance, supposing that the listener is in a joyful mood and wants that mood continued, but the selection is of a sad mood, does this, in any way, interfere with the music creating a change in the existing mood, or with the degree of enjoyment derived from the music ?

9. Which mood change is more enjoyed—from serious to joyful, or *vice versa*.

10. What is the relation of all these factors to the degree of musicalness of the auditors ?

All these problems form links in one continuous chain of the musical response. Each has its effect upon all the others and one cannot be detached from the rest without affecting the whole. Thus, one cannot separate the mood effect from the degree of enjoyment or the degree of enjoyment from the degree of familiarity, or these from the attitude of the hearer towards the

CHART I

SHOWING THE EFFECTS OF MUSIC ON EXISTING MOODS

+ Change.
− No Effect.

OBSERVERS

Selections.	W.B.	D.C.	R.D.	E.D.	E.H.	G.M.	P.M.	G.I.	R.K.	N.K.	L.M.	M.M.	L.P.	F.R.	I.W.	M.L.	M.W.
Humoreske	00 +		2 +	4 +	6 +	2	6 +	6 +	6 +	0 −	4 +	6 +	00 +		2 +	00 +	
May is Here		4 +	6 +		6 +		6 +		6 +	00 +		4 +		0 −	4 +		
Evening Star	4 +		6 +	4 +	4 +	4 +	6 +			4 +	00 +	6 +	4 +	6 +	00 +		
Berceuse			6 +		2 +		6 +			4 +		6 +		6 +	6 +		
Asa's Tod	6 +		6 +	4 +			6 +		4 +	6 +		2 +	2 +	6 +	6 +	6 +	
Funeral March			6 +	4 +	00 +	6 +	6 +	4 +	4 +	6 +	0 −	0 −	2 +	2 +	2 +		
Ave Maria	6 +	4 +	6 +	4 +	4 +	6 +	4 +	4 +	6 +	4 +	00 +	2 +	+	00 +	6 +	6 +	6 +
Kamennoi-Ostrow	4 +		6 +	00 +	00 +	6 +	6 +		6 +	6 +		6 +	00 +	4 +	4 +		
Liebesfreud	6 +		6 +	6 +	6 +	6 +	4 +		6 +	4 +	0 −	6 +	2 +	6 +	4 +		
Pastel-Minuet	6 +	2 +	4 +	4 +	4 +		6 +	4 +	4 +	4 +		2 +	4 +	4 +	6 +	6 +	4 +
Anitra's Dance			6 +	4 +				4 +	4 +	6 +		4 +		2 +	4 +		
Shepherd Dance			6 +	6 +			6 +		6 +	6 +		6 +		4 +	6 +		
Aida March			6 +		4 +		6 +		6 +	4 +	2 +	4 +		4 +	00 +		
Light Cavalry Overture	00 +		6 +	2 +	6 +	4 +	6 +	6 +	6 +	00 +	00 +	6 +	00 +	6 +	00 +		
Tell Overture	6 +		4 +	4 +	6 +	6 +	6 +	6 +	6 +	6 +	00 +	0 −	00 +		00 +	6 +	4 +

particular type of music represented by the selection, since all function together in the act of appreciation and all determine, although in unequal degrees, the general response of the hearer. It was therefore thought best to obtain information upon all these apparently diverse problems in a single act of listening rather than isolate each item for a separate investigation.

In planning the investigation, the following classification of types of music was used :—

1. Dreamy, vague, soothing, tranquil, soft, leisurely.
2. Sentimental, passionate, yearning, pleading, melting, tender.
3. Sad, pathetic, tragic, plaintive, mournful, doleful.
4. Solemn, spiritual, awe-inspiring, sober, deep, grave.
5. Cheerful, fanciful, joyous, gay, playful.
6. Fanciful, graceful, soaring, sprightly, quaint.
7. Spirited, exciting, exhilarating, agitated, impetuous, restless, sparkling, scintillating, vivacious, rippling, sweeping, gliding.
8. Martial, majestic, dignified, stately, dramatic.
9. Sensational, stormy, thrilling.

The music material consisted of the following selections chosen to represent the above types :—

1. Humoresque, Spalding, violin.
   May is Here, orchestra.
2. Evening Star, cello, Gruppe.
   Berceuse, cello, Sandby.
3. Asa's Tod, band.
   Funeral March, Gardner, violin.
4. Ave Maria, Flesch, violin.
   Kamennoi-Ostrow, orchestra.
5. Liebesfreud, Czewonky, violin.
6. Pastel-Minuet, instrumental trio.
   Anitra's Dance, instrumental trio.
7. Shepherd's Dance, orchestra.
8. Light Cavalry Overture, band.
9. William Tell Overture, band.

Broadly all these selections were further grouped into the following two classes according to possible mood effects :—

CHART II

Selections	EXISTING MOODS					MOOD EFFECTS				
	Joyful	Composed	Nervous	Dreamy	Sad	Joyful	Composed	Nervous	Dreamy	Sad
Liebesfreud	1	1	4	2	4	8			3	1
Pastel Minuet	1	5	6	2	3	13	3			1
Anitra's Dance	3	1	3		1	7	1			
Shepherd's Dance	4	2	2		1	8	1	2		
Alda March	3	2	3	1		4	1	1	1	
Light Cavalry	8		3	1	1	12			1	
William Tell	10	1	1	1		10		2	2	
May is Here	1	3	4		1	3	2	2	2	
Humoreske	8		5			2		5	6	6
Evening Star	10	2	1					1	6	6
Berceuse	4	1	2	1		1			5	2
Ave Maria	2	1	10		4		2	1	9	5
Kamenoi Ostrow	2	1	2		7	1	2	3	5	1
Asa's Tod	5	1	2						2	6
Funeral March	3	2	6		1	1		1	1	8

1. Joyful—
   Liebesfreud.
   Pastel-Minuet.
   Anitra's Dance.
   Shepherd's Dance.
   Aida March.
   Light Cavalry Overture.
   William Tell Overture.

2. Serious—
   May is Here.
   Humoresque.
   Evening Star.
   Berceuse.
   Ave Maria
   Kamennoi-Ostrow.
   Asa's Tod.
   Funeral March.

The investigation was limited to instrumental music, since there is reason to believe that vocal music differs somewhat in its effect and should therefore be made the subject for a separate study.

The observers consisted of seventeen men and women, some of them students of the music and drama departments of the Carnegie Institute of Technology, and others of faculty members of the Division of Co-operative Research. Through a personal interview with the investigator an estimate of the relative degree of musicalness of each observer was made. Information about their musical training, experience, musical likes, dislikes and other details throwing light upon their attitude towards music as a whole was obtained by means of a questionnaire. Following the interview and the filling out of the questionnaire each observer listened to the musical selections in the following order :—

1st session—Ave Maria, Pastel-Minuet, William Tell Overture, Humoresque.

2nd session—Light Cavalry Overture, Evening Star, Liebesfreud.

3rd session—Kamennoi-Ostrow, Funeral March.

4th session—May is Here, Berceuse.

5th session—Anitra's Dance, Asa's Tod, Shepherd's Dance.

In grouping the selections an attempt was made to include for each hearing as much variety as possible in order to obtain from each session some data upon each of the problems enumerated. Each observer was given a form like the accompanying illustration on which his reaction to each selection was recorded.

1. State below, as definitely as you can, your general state of being at the present moment, physical, and mental, particularly the *mood* you are in. For example, " I am tired, and feel somewhat depressed, feel like taking a walk or a chat with a friend, need some relaxation, etc."————

2. Do you enjoy the mood you are in at present, or are you eager to change it, or are you indifferent ?————

3. If eager to change the present mood, what kind of mood would you rather be in ?   Comment freely.————

4. You will now hear a piece of music. Put yourself in the same attitude you would adopt at a concert, or, in other words, free your mind of everything and give yourself up entirely to the music. You have absolutely nothing to do now but listen. Do not read what follows.

5. Now do what you did at the very beginning, namely, comment in full on your present mood and state of being. Do not put down anything because you think it will sound nice, but give as accurate a picture of yourself at the present moment as you possibly can————

6. Below are four numbers.   Underscore one of them to indicate the degree of your enjoyment of the music you just heard. 00 means you were irritated by the music, 0 no effect, 2 enjoyed slightly, 4 moderately, 6 greatly.

   00   0   2   4   6

7. Do you judge the selection you just heard as being good or poor music, irrespective of the enjoyment you got from it ?   Underscore your judgment below.

  Very poor, poor, fair, good, very good.

8. What kind of music would you like to hear now, in preference to any other kind ?   Describe it as well as you can————————

——————————————————————————————————

——————————————————————————————————

9. Indicate below your familiarity with the selection you just heard.

  new, slightly familiar, familiar, very familiar.

Give the name of the selection if you can————————

It will be noticed that this form departs radically from other forms intended for the same purpose in several particulars. Firstly, no moods are stated for the observer to underscore, either before or after hearing the music, but instead a free and spontaneous report is called for. To ask a person to underscore one or more words listed, representing a mood, involves more or less the suggesting of a mood, as if to say " which of the following will you have " or " which of the following pleases you most " ? Comparing our results from the first form of the mood chart where moods are enumerated with the results from the second form where no moods are mentioned, we find that the former, although much more convenient for purposes of tabulation, tells but part of the story, and that part incorrectly. Thus, for instance, a free statement from the observer concerning his affective state of being often reveals the presence of more or less conflicting moods fighting for supremacy. In estimating then the effect of the music, it is certainly very important that the experimenter be aware of all the conflicting moods in which the subject finds himself rather than force him to select the mood that seems to be at the surface at any specific moment.

Second, everything that has been said concerning the statement of moods existing before the music is heard also applies to the statement of the mood effects of the music. To illustrate, several of the observers were much annoyed during some of the renditions either by the interpretation given the selection or by the grating of the phonograph disk, so that the effect produced by the music upon these hearers was not due solely to the music, but also to something outside the music. Consequently, to force the persons to limit themselves to a word or two for the description of the effect of the music would fail to tell the whole story and therefore lead to a false interpretation of the data. Furthermore, it is no simple matter for most persons to compress their state of being into one or two words, the result probably being that after a slight effort to do so they either give up the attempt and underscore any word in a flippant manner, or pick out a word that sounds nice, or a word that they think represents the mood. On the other hand, no matter how flippant or careless or lacking in introspective power one may be, it is probable that in writing several sentences aiming at self-analysis one will reveal to the careful experimenter the predominant mood or moods existing at the time of writing. Although then, the method followed in this procedure involves a great deal more labour in tabulating the results, the reward is found in the greater confidence that one can place in the results.

Mood Change

Chart I gives the effect of each selection as reported by each observer, indicating whether the music produced or failed to produce a change in the existing mood. The plus sign signifies a change, the minus sign no effect. The latter means that the music failed to arouse a reaction in the observer of sufficient intensity to make him conscious either of a change of mood or of an intensification of the existing mood. The figures adjacent to the plus and minus signs indicate the degree of enjoyment for each selection for each observer.

The occurrence of no effect (o) is so rare as to be negligible for practical purposes, while from the statements of those reporting oo, it is evident that the irritation was due, in the majority of cases, to manner of interpretation (playing out of tune, grating, poor tonal quality, dragging, etc.) and in the rest of the cases to a dislike for a particular type of music, instruments, or instrumental combinations. Thus, for instance, the " Humoresque " annoyed most of the listeners because the recording was very badly out of tune, the most musical of the observers stating this specifically, while many stated that there was something wrong with the selection. Again, in the case of " Kamennoi-Ostrow ", the rendition is dragged out and the composition mutilated by omissions, the observers reporting the first item specifically, and the second by vaguer statements of there being something wrong with the piece. In the " Light Cavalry Overture " the irritation was produced by the unpleasant quality of the instruments, the trombones, in particular, emitting ear-splitting tones. The " Evening Star ", another selection, resulting in many oo's, is given a very unmusical interpretation, although played by one of the foremost 'cellists of the day.

Eliminating, then, the few cases of no effect, as irrelevant in the present case the chart indicates definitely that the selections used in this study produced a change of mood in every instance in the seventeen listeners or intensified an existing mood when in conformity with the mood of the music, both effects giving some degree of enjoyment.

Uniformity of Mood Effect

The power of music to change an existing mood is perhaps neither as interesting nor as significant as the degree of uniformity of mood induced by the same selection in all hearers. In Chart II the mood distribution of the listeners before and after hearing the music is shown. The moods included under each key word are the same for this chart as for Chart I.

Of the moods before the music for the seven selections in Class I (joyful), thirty are in agreement with the music, while fifty-four are in moods contrary to that of the music. Of the moods after the music for the same group of selection sixty-two are in moods similar to that of the music and sixteen in moods differing from that of the music. Of these sixteen contrary moods, we note that three report irritation, which, as previously mentioned, is due not to the music so much as to the manner of rendition. (Wherever a discrepancy occurs in the number of moods before and moods after the music, it is due to the failure of some of the observers to report the effect of some of the selections.) Of the seventy-two moods before the music for the *calm-restful, dreamy-pensive* classes of selections nine are in agreement with the music, and sixty-three different from the music ; while of the seventy-two induced moods, thirty-nine fall under the moods inherent in the music. Of the remaining thirty-three, fourteen report irritation and nervousness, due to rendition, or dislike for a type of music, and fourteen fall under the *sad* class, a mood which few persons could differentiate from the *dreamy-*

pensive class. Of the twenty pre-audition moods for the *depressed-sad* class of music, one agrees with the music and nineteen are contrary, while of the nineteen post-audition moods, fourteen agree with the music, one reports nervousness and three belong in the *dreamy-pensive* class.

Summarizing the data from Charts I and II, we conclude that the large variety of selections used in this investigation, produced not only a change of mood in practically all the listeners, but also that the moods induced by each selection, or the same class of selections, as reported by the large majority of our hearers, are strikingly similar in type.

To obtain further evidence and in greater detail on the consistency of musical effect, data were obtained from a large number of listeners who heard ten selections under the same circumstances at two separate times. The purpose was to see whether the hearers would record the same effect the second time that they reported on the first hearing.[1]

The material selected for this experiment consisted of ten phonograph selections. Five of these were instrumental and five vocal numbers. The selections were chosen on the basis of previous study to represent different types of music and musical effects. It was intended that physical, emotional, imaginative, and ideational responses should be included. The selections used were as follows :—

> Stars and Stripes For Ever.
> Menuetto All' Anti'co.
> Blue Danube Waltz.
> To a Wild Rose.
> At the Brook.
>
> Anvil Chorus.
> He Shall Feed His Flock.
> Les Oiseaux dans la Charmille.
> Love's Old Sweet Song.
> Ave Maria.

[1] This part of the investigation was conducted by Mr. Gatewood.

The observers in this experiment were college girls. Fifty-three attended the first programme, forty-seven the second programme seventeen days later. Thirty-two heard both and on their reports this study is based. The conditions were kept as natural as possible. At seven-thirty in the evening when everything else at Camp had become quiet the girls came together. They sat comfortably around the instrument, listening to the selections for pleasure. A record blank like the accompanying illustration was provided for each observer. At the close of each number, each observer checked the

---

How do you feel ?   Indicate by check mark.

happy	tired	discouraged
sad	rested	excited
bright	worried	serious
dull	depressed	restless

What kind of music do you feel like hearing ?   Check one or more

gay	bright	dreamy	stimulating
solemn	dull	martial	quieting
joyous	tender	religious	sentimental
sad	majestic	humorous	

After each selection, note how it made you feel and record by a check mark in the appropriate spaces :—

Effect on you.						Selections.									
						1	2	3	4	5	6	7	8	9	10
Happy	.	.	.	.	.										
Sad	.	.	.	.	.										
Gay	.	.	.	.	.										
Serious	.	.	.	.	.										
Amused	.	.	.	.	.										
Felt like dancing	.	.	.	.	.										
Rested	.	.	.	.	.										
Irritated	.	.	.	.	.										
Physically stirred	.	.	.	.											
Feeling of majesty	.	.	.	.											
Tender memories	.	.	.	.											
Imagination and fancy	.	.	.	.											
Devotional mood	.	.	.	.											
Feeling of patriotism	.	.	.	.											
Longing	.	.	.	.	.										
Sentimental	.	.	.	.											
Was it familiar ?	.	.	.	.											

Which selection did you like best ? ....
            least ? ....
Date................................. Time ....
Name ....
Address ....

term or terms which described the way the selection
made her feel. Much interest was shown throughout
the experiment and a wholly serious report was received.

The number of observers who recorded at the second
hearing of a selection the same feeling which they
recorded at the first hearing is surprisingly large. In
terms of percentage of observers, the numbers for each
selection are as follows :—

PER CENT OF OBSERVERS RECORDING THE SAME
EFFECT ON SECOND HEARING AS ON FIRST.

Numbers.	Per Cent.
Les Oiseaux dans la Charmille . .	91
Anvil Chorus	80
Stars and Stripes For Ever . . .	77
Love's Old Sweet Song. . . .	64
To a Wild Rose	62
He Shall Feed His Flock . . .	60
At the Brook	59
Blue Danube Waltz	53
Ave Maria	50
Menuetto All' Anti'co	45

These figures are significant. Only one selection,
"Menuetto All' Anti'co," gave the same effect to less
than fifty per cent of the observers on second hearing.
With sixteen different possible effects we should expect
some very low percentages. By laws of chance, the
probability that a person would select the same effect
a second time is one-sixteenth. The probability of each
person's selecting the same effect is so small that the high
percentages become very significant. It means that a
definite reaction is stimulated. The intrinsic quality
of the music must be such as to arouse the same physiological response. Certain outside factors, such as the
mood which the listener brings to the concert, the
memories or associations aroused, and certain experimental factors will vary from time to time, so that many
variations do occur, but a marked consistency is present.

L

Comparison of the most dominant effect, i.e., the effect recorded by the greatest number in the first hearing, and the most dominant effect reported in the second hearing gives to us further evidence of consistency. The leading effects are as follows :—

Number.	First Hearing.	Second Hearing.
Stars and Stripes For Ever .	Physically stirred	Physically stirred.
Menuetto All' Anti'co . .	Imagination and fancy	Imagination and fancy (rested).
Blue Danube Waltz . .	Dancing	Dancing.
To a Wild Rose . . .	Rested	Longing.
At the Brook . . .	Imagination and fancy	Imagination and fancy.
Anvil Chorus . . .	Physically stirred	Physically stirred.
He Shall Feed His Flock .	Irritated	Irritated.
Les Oiseaux dans la Charmille	Amused	Amused.
Love's Old Sweet Song. .	Tender memories	Tender memories (longing).
Ave Maria	Serious	Rested.

With only two exceptions the leading effect is the same in both instances. The change in these two is not great. In the one, " To a Wild Rose," *rested* and *longing* are the two leading effects. The one is predominantly a physical condition, whereas the other is predominantly a mental condition, neither one exclusive of the other. In the first hearing almost as many observers recorded *longing* as *rested,* so that the change of only two observers' judgments shifted the relative position of the two effects. In " Ave Maria " *serious* and *rested* are the two leading effects. In the first hearing *rested* was recorded by only one less observer than *serious,* hence a slight shift in individual judgments caused a shift in relative position of these effects. Both effects were recorded by many as neither effect in any way excludes the other. In fact, that music which calms and rests one is most apt to be that which arouses serious contemplation.

Among the ten selections, eight are characterized as different on the basis of dominant or leading effect. Many other incidental effects are recorded which contributed, no doubt, in large measure to the total effect of the music. The fact that eight different leading effects were designated indicates that the a priori selection of disparate types was sufficiently accurate.

TOTAL NUMBER OF APPEARANCES OF EACH EFFECT

Rested . . .	106	Happy . . .	56
Imagination and fancy .	102	Sad	51
Irritated . . .	87	Dancing . . .	43
Amused . . .	84	Patriotic . . .	36
Physically stirred .	77	Sentimental . .	33
Serious . . .	74	Gay	32
Longing . . .	68	Majestic . . .	30
Memories . . .	59	Devotional . .	23

These figures represent the number of times any given effect is recorded throughout the concert. For example, the feeling of *rest* was reported 106 times. It is a significant fact that with one exception the eight effects which stood out as leading effects are the eight highest on the basis of total occurrences. This means that as incidental effects they are also most frequently aroused. They are the effects most frequently experienced as a result of listening to music. The one exception, dancing, is a very decided one, inasmuch as music of this character forms a large group in itself. The effect of listening to music of the dance type is largely physical. The inherent rhythm, tempo, and volume are such that they bring out increased physiological responses. Music of slower tempo, less decided accent, and with easy flowing melody results in slower physiological response. It is these selections, giving the feeling of rest that are often accompanied by ideational and imaginative processes.

The proportion of music which has an irritating effect is very small. It so happens that the one pyrotechnic record included was very irritating to many and especially so to a group of girls which did not understand the technique with which it is accomplished. Practically only two effects, amused and irritated, were recorded. There was not the usual distribution of incidental or secondary effects.

It is a significant fact that imagination or fancy is scored high in those records which show low consistency and does not appear at all in the records showing high consistency. It is evidently a variable effect, dependent largely on represented factors, i.e. not from the music itself, but from conditions and associations peculiar to the individual himself. When some one effect is consistently aroused, imaginative effects are not prominent.

As incidental effect, the relative order of frequency of the several effects is somewhat different from that in which count is made of the total number of occurrences. By subtracting the number of times in which an effect is scored as the dominant effect from the total number of its occurrences, a measure of the secondary or contributing importance of the various effects is obtained. The order for the two varies considerably. However, in the upper eight of each series, six of the effects are the same, namely, *rested, serious, physically stirred, longing, imagination and fancy, memories.* It is particularly significant that *rest* ranks first in both cases. *Devotion* is sixteenth in total scores and fifteenth in secondary scoring. The correlation of the two rankings is sixty-three. *Happy* and *sad* are two incidental or secondary effects which occur with marked frequency. The very high position of *irritating* in this set of selections is not substantiated by other trials. It is out of its due position here, owing to the fact that one particular record, " Les Oiseaux dans la Charmille ", gave but two effects, practically (amusement and irritation) which in a small group of this sort gives it undue weight.   The more logical order becomes :—

> Rested.
> Happy.
> Serious.
> Sad.
> Physically stirred.
> Longing.
> Imagination and fancy.
> Memories.
> Patriotic.

On what effects is there the greatest agreement ?   In other words, where there is a well-marked effect, dominant in both hearings, which quality or effect is agreed upon by the greatest number ?   This relative order is represented as follows :—

Selection.	Rank.	Effect.
Les Oiseaux dans la Charmille .	1	Amusement.
Stars and Stripes For Ever . .	2	Physically stirred.
He Shall Feed His Flock . .	3	Irritated.
Menuetto All' Anti'co . . .	4	Imagination and fancy.
At the Brook	5·5	Imagination and fancy.
Anvil Chorus	5·5	Physically stirred.
Blue Danube Waltz . . .	7·5	Dancing.
Love's Old Sweet Song. . .	7·5	Tender memories.
Ave Maria.	9	Serious—to rested.
To a Wild Rose	10	Rested—to longing.

The selection which ranks highest, " Les Oiseaux dans la Charmille ", is an unusual case, and is perhaps not as representative a selection as are the others.   However, that there is marked agreement on the amusing effect, when present, is very evident.   This does not mean that the effect of amusing selections is more intense, but rather that where the amusing quality is the leading effect, it is felt by practically all hearers.   At least three factors enter in : (1) the effect, (2) efficacy of the record, (3) representative material.

The first means that certain feelings are inherently more generally experienced than others. These are those to which some writers refer as elemental effects. For instance, a feeling of longing is not apt to be aroused in each one of a group as readily as is the tendency to dance or the feeling of amusement, other things being equal. A considerable amount of variation is found due to the record itself. For example, a poorly made record of a hymn, which under favourable circumstances would inspire a decided feeling of devotion, might arouse only a feeling of irritation or perhaps of amusement. Furthermore, the attitude and the mood with which each hearer listens, his own personal experiences which are in some ways unlike those of anyone else, his associations—these and other personal factors cause variations in final effect. The total effect is derived from two factors, the presented material, which is the actual music itself, and the represented material, which of necessity varies. The fact that certain selections may arouse such similar representative material is even more singular.

CONCLUSIONS

The data show that the same effects are experienced upon hearing a selection at different times. In other words, there is a marked consistency in the response which music arouses.

The dominant effect, or that which most observers agree to be the leading effect from a selection, is the same when the selection is heard at different times.

On the basis of this group of musical selections a feeling of *rest* is the most frequent result. This seems to hold generally true of arm-chair music, which makes up the library of a vast proportion of music-loving persons.

Amusing and physically stirring selections evoke the greatest amount of agreement among hearers on the basis of leading effect. This probably means that where these factors are dominant in the selection, all hearers report the same effect more often than when other factors are the dominant ones.

Introspective report shows reliability sufficient to more than justify its use in the study of the effects of music, particularly where the results from a large number of observers are desired. The fact that after a period of many days, without any reference to the previous programme and its results, so large a per cent of the hearers record the same effect which they recorded the previous time evidences the fact that the music actually arouses a definite effect. Some music is more definite in the responses it arouses than is other music. Most music will call up secondary or related feelings dependent largely on the individual differences of the listeners' mood and experience. No two people are affected exactly the same by any stimulus. The study shows, however, that a given musical selection will arouse a certain definite reaction and will arouse the same reaction on different occasions. in a large proportion of those who listen.

CHAPTER VIII

PROBLEMS RELATED TO THE MOOD EFFECTS OF MUSIC

MAX SCHOEN AND ESTHER L. GATEWOOD

1. *Feelings and Emotions resulting from Music as a Stimulus* [1]

WHICH emotional qualities are most frequently aroused by music ? Is music effective in arousing all kinds of feelings ? Certain of the emotional effects which are very common in everyday life are rarely if ever aroused by music alone. Anger for example, is one of the most instinctive tendencies, and genetically functions very early in life. However, the nature of music is such that there are certain limitations to the sort of effect that may result from it. It is difficult to conceive of a person becoming very angry from the hearing of music. He may become angry at certain circumstances accompanying the performance—some distracting noises, as, for instance, talking in the audience, or he may become angry on account of remembering circumstances connected with a previous hearing of the musical selection, or its words may arouse memories of experiences of his own past which may re-arouse a feeling of anger. But the music alone would never make one really angry.

What then are the feelings that music incites most frequently ?

In a preliminary experiment, the recording sheet included some effects which were seldom if ever reported

[1] This study is based on the data from the experiment reported in Chapter IV.

by the listeners. In the present study these were omitted, but the listeners endeavoured on all occasions to record, and make special note of any effects, feelings, or emotions, resulting from the music which were not indicated on the recording sheet. None were reported, so that it becomes safe to conclude that the eleven listed below are the effects usually derived from listening to music.

In a list of five hundred and eighty-nine selections, practically all types of music are represented. This does not mean that all types are represented in equal proportions, but it is likely that the relative proportions within these five hundred and eighty-nine selections is very near that of music, at least phonograph music, in general.

Eleven emotional effects occur in the records. The relative frequencies of these eleven are determined in the following manner. If each listener reported a certain effect from each selection, a total of one thousand seven hundred and sixty-seven records would be the result. This represents the greatest number of times any item could occur. Using this figure then as the common denominator, the actual frequencies of appearance of the various emotional qualities were converted into relative frequencies.

RELATIVE FREQUENCY OF APPEARANCE OF
VARIOUS EMOTIONAL EFFECTS

Emotional Quality.	No. of Appear.	Relative Frequency.
Rest . . .	698	·39
Sadness . . .	798	·45
Joy	728	·41
Love . . .	628	·35
Longing . . .	535	·30
Amusement . .	229	·12
Dignity . . .	349	·20
Stirring . . .	501	·28
Reverence . .	243	·14
Disgust . . .	37	·02
Irritation . . .	160	·08

Using the total number of times any emotional effect was marked, four thousand nine hundred and six, the relative proportions of the various emotional items are as follows :—

PROPORTION OF EACH EMOTIONAL EFFECT IN
TERMS OF TOTAL SCORINGS OF EMOTIONAL
EFFECTS

Emotional Quality.	No. of Appear.	Propor. Frequency.
Rest . . .	698	14
Sadness . . .	798	16
Joy	728	15
Love . . .	628	13
Longing . . .	535	11
Amusement . .	229	5
Dignity . . .	349	7
Stirring . . .	501	10
Reverence . .	243	5
Disgust . .	37	1
Irritation . . .	160	3

The rank order for the several emotions is the same on the basis of proportional frequency and on the basis of relative frequency. Proportional frequency is an expression in terms of the number of times an emotional effect of any sort appeared, whereas relative frequency is in terms of the number of times which a given effect *might* have been reported.

Sadness is reported as a result of music more than any other one effect. *Joy*, however, is reported in almost as many instances, and *rest* only slightly less than *joy*. These three, together with *love, longing* and *stirring*, are the pronounced effects which result from listening to music. *Amusement, dignity* and *reverence*, although in small proportions, are clearly evident effects, when one remembers that the intrinsic nature of these effects is such as to depend on a limited group of musical selections.

Some differences in the relative frequency with which all reports agreed upon the several effects is evident.

How many selections were reported to arouse a given effect in each hearer alike ? The following tables show the relative frequency of each emotional quality, when recorded by each judge, and *show* also the differences which exist in the relative proportions of each quality in selections of high emotional character and those of low emotional character.

TABLE OF RELATIVE FREQUENCY OF UNIFORMITY OF EFFECT

Class I

Emotional Quality.	No. of Appear.	% of Group (261).	% whole (589).
Rest .	59	22	10
Sadness	51	20	8·7
Joy .	58	22	10
Love .	61	23	12
Longing	39	15	6·8
Amusement	8	3	1·4
Dignity	9	3·5	1·5
Stirring	40	15	6·8
Reverence .	23	8·8	3·8

TABLE OF RELATIVE FREQUENCY OF UNIFORMITY OF EFFECT

Class II

Emotional Quality.	No. of Appear.	% of Group (173).	% whole (589).
Rest .	33	19	5·6
Sadness	67	39	11·4
Joy .	63	36	10·6
Love .	9	11	3·2
Longing	12	7	2
Amusement	29	17	5
Dignity	9	5	1·5
Stirring	30	17	5
Reverence .	7	4	1·2

While *joy, rest* and *sadness* still rank very high in frequency when only these instances in which all observers' reports agreed are considered, in Class I, where the quantitative estimate is greater than average, the emotional quality occurring most often is *love*. This means that when a pronounced feeling of *love* is aroused, it is definite and experienced by several alike, whereas *rest, sadness* and *joy*, while showing great consistency, are in some measure more variable, more flexible than the more limited feelings of *love, longing, amusement, reverence*, and so forth. A musical selection may give *joy* to one person, *sadness* to another, and at the same time, by means of the words or some characteristic of the music, arouse a feeling of *longing*. The factor of memories is one which here plays a large rôle. The immediately present stimulus may call forth a reaction of a sort which is alike to all hearers, but the representative (imaginative or memory) material may greatly change some other effects experienced.

Among those selections which give a definite effect but not very marked, *joy* and *sadness* are prominent, *joy* appearing 32 per cent of the time. This is not inconsistent with the proportions of Class I.

When the total emotional effect is very clear, the various hearers' records agree upon the more specific or limited effect. When the emotional effect is less clear, they agree upon the more general effect. By general I do not mean that *joy, sadness* and *rest* do not have definable characteristics, but they are concomitants of the various other effects in many instances. One may be very much rested by a selection that arouses *longing*, one that arouses *love*, or *dignity*, or *reverence*, or even *amusement*. Similarly there are so many sources of *joy* that this feeling may exist together with any one of several other feelings.

Consistency

Thus far we have been speaking only of the relative proportion of different emotional effects in the whole musical group. Quite another problem is that of consistency of effect in many listeners. Which emotional quality shows the most uniformity or is most often recorded by all ?

In the following table the first column of figures represents the number of times each effect was recorded by all three judges. These figures are then converted into terms of consistency by multiplying each figure by three and dividing the product by the total number of times that quality appeared on the data records. For example, rest was recorded by all three ninety-two times. Its total number of appearances was 698.

Its relative consistency then becomes ·40.

TABLE SHOWING RELATIVE CONSISTENCY OF THE SEVERAL QUALITIES IN EFFECT ON SEVERAL HEARERS

Emotional Quality.	No. of times agreed upon.	Relative Cons.
Rest	92	·40
Sadness	118	·44
Joy	121	·50
Love	80	·38
Longing	51	·29
Amusement . . .	37	·48
Dignity	18	·15
Stirring	70	·42
Reverence . . .	30	·37
Disgust	0	0
Irritation . . .	3	·05

The figures are very significant. While it might seem from the data that there was a great deal of variation of effect and one might be led to conclude that there is no reliability as to the effect received from the music, when converted thus into terms of relative consistency quite the contrary becomes evident.

If every time joy was reported, it was so reported by each person, a consistency of one would be obtained. With many elements, which we call representative material, influencing the total stimulus, the effect naturally varies according to the experience of the individual. Certain memories are aroused by this or that portion of the music, the instrumentation, its rhythm, etc. In spite of these very vital forces in the total effect derived from listening to music, the consistency is very marked for most of the recorded effects. *Joy, amusement, sadness, stirring, rest, love* and *reverence*, show particularly high consistency. More than that they show a similar degree of uniformity, which is indicative of the effectiveness of music in arousing definite emotional effects in many listeners.

2. *A Comparison of Instrumental and Vocal Music as Stimulants to Emotional Effect*

Even those who admit that certain kinds of music may have a definite effect, limit those kinds largely to vocal music, where the words convey the meaning to the listeners and arouse memory images in much the same manner as the recounting of a story or a familiar description. Our study has definitely shown that instrumental music does give well-defined and consistent emotional effects. But does instrumental music give as well-marked and uniform effects as vocal music ?

The following table gives the numbers and the percentages of instrumental and vocal selections belonging in each class, according to effect. Class I includes those selections from which all hearers reported the same effect and that to a marked degree ; Class II, selections of uniform effect, but not to marked degree ; Class III, selections of diverse effect, but of marked degree ; Class IV, selections of neither consistency of effect, nor of marked effect.

Group.	Instrumental.		Vocal.	
	Number.	Per cent.	Number.	Per cent.
I	93	38	168	48
II	74	30·5	99	29
III	13	5	20	6
IV	65	26·5	57	17
Total	245		344	

For ten per cent more vocal numbers than instrumental numbers clearly defined emotional effects of marked degree (Class I) are reported. Class II and Class III show practically no difference in the relative proportions of instrumental and vocal selections. Class IV, on the other hand, shows exactly the reverse of Class I, having ten per cent more instrumental numbers than vocal.

Much greater consistency of judgment is found in vocal than in instrumental selections. The relative consistency of the two is shown in the following figures :

	Total No. Selections.	Agree. Abo. ave. in degree.	Agree. Below ave. in degree.	Total No. times consistent.
Vocal . . .	344	239	175	414
Instrumental . .	245	98	97	195

The proportion of vocal selections on which all hearers agreed as to emotional quality is very much higher than that of instrumental selections. Moreover, in those cases which show agreement the quantitative measurements show that a more uniform effect is reported from vocal than from instrumental music. In instrumental selections there is an equal distribution between high and low degrees of emotional quality.

Vocal music, due unquestionably to the words, has greater power to arouse a definite emotional response than has instrumental music. Some emotional feeling is dependent upon thoughts largely. Which emotions are most dependent upon the words of a song is shown by means of a comparison of the relative percentages of vocal and instrumental selections for each emotional quality.

TABLE SHOWING RELATIVE PROPORTIONS OF INSTRUMENTAL AND VOCAL MUSIC AROUSING THE VARIOUS AFFECTIVE QUALITIES

Class I

	INSTRUMENTAL.				VOCAL.		
	Number.	% (on basis of class).	% (on basis of whole group).		Number.	% (on basis of class).	% (on basis of whole group).
Rest . .	29	27·5	12		30	12	8·7
Sadness .	11	10	4·5		40	17	11·4
Joy . .	33	31·5	13		25	10	7·3
Love . .	2	2	·8		59	24	17·2
Longing .	4	4	1·6		35	14	10
Amusement	0	0	0		8	3	2·3
Dignity .	4	4	1·6		5	2	1·5
Stirring .	22	21	9		18	7·5	5·2
Reverence .	0	0	0		23	10	6·7
	105				243		

Class II

	INSTRUMENTAL.				VOCAL.		
	Number.	% (on basis of class).	% (on basis of whole group).		Number.	% (on basis of class).	% (on basis of whole group).
Rest . .	14	12	5·6		19	13	5·5
Sadness .	30	25	12·2		37	25	10·5
Joy . .	43	35	17·6		20	13	5·9
Love . .	6	5	2·4		13	9	3·8
Longing .	6	5	2·4		6	4	1·8
Amusement	6	5	2·4		23	16	6·7
Dignity .	4	3	1·6		5	3	1·5
Stirring .	12	10	4·9		18	12	5·2
Reverence .	0	0	0		7	5	2
	121				148		

The percentages of the whole instrumental group may be directly compared with the percentages of the whole vocal group. Converted into ratio terms the relative proportions of instrumental and vocal music producing the several effects to a high degree are as follows :—

TABLE SHOWING RATIO OF INSTRUMENTAL AND
VOCAL MUSIC GIVING EACH EFFECT

Class I

	Instrumental.	Vocal.
Rest . . .	1·3	1
Sadness . . .	1	3
Joy	2	1
Love . . .	1	17
Longing . . .	1	5
Amusement . .	0	2
Dignity . . .	1	1
Stirring . . .	1	5
Reverence . .	0	7

These figures mean that three times as many vocal numbers as instrumental were reported to arouse a feeling of *sadness* ; two times as many instrumental numbers as vocal were reported to arouse a feeling of *joy*, and so forth.

So far as one may conclude from this number of musical selections, *rest* results about equally from instrumental and vocal music.

The feeling of *dignity* is aroused equally by both kinds of music. *Sadness, love, longing, amusement, stirring* and *reverence* seem undoubtedly to be the results of vocal music more than of instrumental, while *joy* is the result of instrumental music twice as often as from vocal.

Among those musical selections which show evident but less marked effects less striking ratios exist, but in no instance is the tendency different from that shown in the figures of Class I. In other words, in no instance where vocal music is more effective in stimulating a given response to a marked degree, does instrumental music show greater effectiveness when the response is less marked. Though the relative proportions are not as striking as in Class I, the figures substantiate rather than contradict the earlier data.

TABLE SHOWING RATIO OF INSTRUMENTAL AND
VOCAL MUSIC GIVING EACH EFFECT

Class II

	Instrumental.	Vocal.
Rest	1	1
Sadness	1·1	1
Joy	3	1
Love	1	2
Longing	1	1
Amusement	1	4
Dignity	1	1
Stirring	1	1
Reverence	0	2

The greater efficacy is in the same direction whether the emotional effect is merely definite or of marked degree. It is quite natural to expect the ratios to be more striking in the latter case. Many selections of either sort may show any one of the several qualities, and yet not give a strong emotional appeal.

While the fact that none of the instrumental selections were reported to arouse a feeling of reverence does not mean that such an effect is never thus created, it does show that this effect depends largely upon the expression of some idea or thought by means of the words of a song. Such instrumental music as is reported to arouse a devotional attitude had probably been heard at some time with sacred words or is reminiscent of sacred music. This does not deny the usefulness of a certain type of instrumental music in church or other devotional services. Such music is most valuable, but its influence lies in the creation of other states, such as rest, which are closely related to the state of *reverence*. Relaxation, or freedom from worrying thoughts, is the foundation of a reverential attitude. Quieting music and softened light are two of the most potent factors in producing this state. But rarely does instrumental music possess the power of directly producing *reverence* or *devotion*. Vocal music of the appropriate sort is much more potent.

Amusement is another response which is the source of much pleasure derived from music, and which is largely dependent upon vocal music. Humorous descriptions, ridiculous words, peculiarities of voice and manner, are the most striking means of amusing people through music. Certain incongruities and amusing effects are well obtained by means of instruments, as for example, " The Elephant and the Fly " and " Make that Trombone Laugh ". Such selections are particularly interesting to children and represent a much more wholesome type of entertainment than most comic songs.

Love and *longing* are both predominantly effects resulting from vocal music. The factor just mentioned in another connexion, namely words and the meaning thereby conveyed, is very potent in arousing the feelings of *love* and *longing*. There are in addition two other factors of importance. The first of these is memory or association. A love song when it is first heard appeals to experiences or feelings within the hearer similar to those embodied in the song. Then, when such a song is again heard, these same memories return and heighten the emotional effect. Both of these types of music are peculiarly personal. References to mother, home, sweetheart, children, or native land have an intimate personal meaning for each listener, and arouse correspondingly intimate emotional feeling.

The second factor is the characteristic nature of the music used in these two types of songs. The simple melody of love songs is peculiarly fitting to that emotion. Similarly of *longing*. That no small portion of the effect is due to the music itself is evident from the fact that in a large number of songs in a foreign tongue, where the words were not at all understood, the music, plus the expression of the singer's voice, aroused these feelings of *love* and *longing*. This simple melodic structure seldom occurs without words. But where it is found, a corresponding emotion is reported, as for example, in " Sweet Spirit Hear My Prayer " by Wallace, or the Pierne " Serenade ".

Joy, on the other hand, is a feeling which finds expression in increased activity, a desire for movement, whether real or ideational. Instrumental music, with its greater flexibility, greater speed and intricate movement is a more adequate stimulus to joy than is vocal music. Certain vocal music has such characteristics and it is these qualities plus the expression of the voice itself which give the feeling of *joy* from songs. The words are of only minor importance, for in many instances where the words are unintelligible or where only vowel tones are used the effect of *joy* is quite as pronounced, as for example, in David's " Charmant Oiseau " .

Sadness, one of the most frequent emotional effects reported from music, is related to vocal music even more than to instrumental. In each one of those selections showing three marked emotional qualities, *sadness* is one of the three, and in one-third of those showing two marked qualities, *sadness* is one. As in the expression of love and longing, the intonation of the human voice is the most potent means of arousing sadness. Here, too, the very legato, quiet melody of sad or melancholy songs becomes tedious when no words accompany it. The tendency of one who feels intense *love* or *sorrow* is to tell someone else, and the human voice becomes both the best means of expression and the most adequate means of arousing these feelings.

Rest is aroused alike by instrumental and vocal music.

Some voices seem to be more suited to this effect than others. For example, very few soprano numbers appear in the list of selections designated as being restful. Low mellow voices seem preferable. For *joy*, on the other hand, flexible soprano voices are desirable. There is a conspicuous absence of percussion instruments in this group. Solos on violin or 'cello, string quartets, and orchestra music more often produce *relaxation* and *rest*.

SUMMARY

Generally speaking, emotions and moods are more often reported as the result of vocal music than of instrumental music. A greater consistency of effect upon several hearers is found with vocal music than with instrumental. However, in the arousal of certain effects, namely, *dignity*, *rest* and *joy*, instrumental music as often or more frequently is the appropriate stimulus. The particular quality of the human voice, the instinctive mode of expression of certain emotions, and the introduction of specific ideas through the words of songs are the chief factors determining the differences in emotional effect between vocal and instrumental music. However, instrumental music may arouse quite as definite and quite as intense emotional responses as vocal music.

3. *The Relation of the Listener's Attitude to the Kind of Music Desired and to the Effect produced by the Music*

The purpose of this study was to investigate the relation of the mood of the hearer to (1) the kind of music which he wished to hear, and (2) to the effect of the given music upon him. What influence does the existing mood have upon the music desired and is this relation constant ?   Is the effect of the music upon the listener influenced by his attitude at the time of listening ?

The original data sheet which was used in the experiment on " A Study in the Consistency of Musical Effect ",[1] asked the listener to record first how he felt, or his present mood, and second what kind of music he desired to hear. Both questions were answered by checking the given set of terms which were descriptive of a variety of moods. The list contained twelve terms.   All the different feelings which we describe are different phases of a dynamic scale varying from a minus quantity to a positive quantity. At the middle point we represent a dynamic balance, a condition of rest wherein the person feels neither a tendency to exert force upon the objective world about him nor does he feel that the objective world is at that moment exerting force upon him.   Those terms which characterize the happy, bright, excited, restless condition, in other words, a surplus of energy desiring an outlet, we shall designate as active.   Those terms then which characterize a depressed, worried, serious, discouraged, dull, sad, tired state, we shall designate as passive.   In reality the second group should be divided into two, distinguishing the merely passive condition in the individual from a depressed condition.   But for our purposes the dual distinction, active and passive, is sufficient.

The descriptive terms given in Question I are therefore divided as follows :—

Active.	Passive.
Happy.	Serious.
Bright.	Sad.
Excited.	Dull.
Restless.	Tired.
	Worried.
	Depressed.
	Discouraged.

[1] Chapter VII, p. 144.

Similarly the terms of Question II characterize two directions of dynamic changes. Just as we have an active feeling, so we have music which is active in its effect. It tends to increase physiological energy. On the other hand is a large group of music which tends to decrease physiological energy. The fifteen terms given to the listeners in Question II can therefore be grouped thus :—

Dynamic.	Quieting.
Gay.	Solemn.
Joyous.	Sad.
Bright.	Dull.
Majestic.	Tender.
Martial.	Dreamy.
Humorous.	Religious.
Stimulating.	Quieting.
	Sentimental.

The second group represents the music which does not call for bodily responses on the part of the listener, whereas the first group represents the music which energizes and stimulates bodily activity.

Present Mood.	Music Desired.		Relation to Existing Mood.	
	Dynamic.	Quieting.	Like.	Unlike.
Happy . . .	40	13	40	13
Tired . . .	23	24	24	23
Serious . .	9	12	12	9
Bright . .	9	4	9	4
Dull . . .	4	4	4	4
Rested . .	3	1	3	1
Worried . .	3	3	3	3
Depressed . .	—	7	7	—
Discouraged .	1	2	2	1
Excited . .	12	5	12	5
Serious . .	9	11	11	9
Restless . .	5	6	5	6
	118	92	132	78

In answer to Question I, there were ninety-four expressions of active mood and one hundred and sixteen of passive. These figures include the several terms used by some listeners. In answer to Question II, an expression of the music desired, there were one hundred and eighteen dynamic terms scored, and ninety-two quieting ones, so that this group of listeners showed somewhat more of a desire for energizing than for quieting music. There are one hundred and thirty-two scores for music dynamically like the existing mood and seventy-eight for music unlike the existing mood.

Where music similar to the existing mood is desired, is it usually in the dynamic or the passive? Among the ninety-four active moods there were sixty-six expressions of a desire for active music (like). Among the one hundred and sixteen passive moods there were sixty-six expressions of desire for passive music (like). The proportion of active wanting active music is greater than passive wanting passive music. But more than half, even of the passive, desire music like the existing mood. The conclusion must be that more people want music in keeping with their feeling at the time than music of contrasting effect.

Is a person's response consistent? For how many people is there a consistent relationship between mood and desired music? How many people want music like their present mood or else always want music unlike the existing mood? Two trials are not enough from which to draw general conclusions. However, on the basis of thirty-two persons who heard both programmes only seven showed a variation in this respect. The remaining twenty-five showed a consistent relationship. If they chose music like the existing mood on one occasion they also did the second time. If, on the other hand, they chose music unlike the existing mood they again chose music unlike the existing mood. It therefore seems to be an individual variation which is consistent with the individual.

The question then arises : How does the same music affect those of different mood ? A comparison was made of the effect of each selection on those who characterized themselves as active and those who characterized themselves as passive. The relative proportions of each group expressing dynamic effects and those expressing depressing effects does not vary. The following table shows the distribution within each group :—

Selection.	ACTIVE AT START.		PASSIVE AT START.	
	Positive effect.	Depressing effect.	Positive effect.	Depressing effect.
Stars and Stripes For Ever . .	31	1	31	5
Menuetto All' Anti'co . . .	9	24	8	25
Blue Danube Waltz . . .	20	16	16	22
To a Wild Rose	0	31	0	39
Spring Song (Mendelssohn) . .	15	20	18	20
Anvil Chorus	30	5	34	3
He Shall Feed His Flock . .	18	15	13	28
Les Oiseaux dans la Charmille .	35	0	40	1
Love's Old Sweet Song . .	4	32	3	37
Ave Maria (Bach-Gounod) (Soprano)	1	33	0	41

Only one selection, " Blue Danube Waltz," shows any decided difference. In this instance, more of the active group reported an active effect and more in the passive group reported a passive effect. The two decided movements in the music itself may explain this difference. This selection is, however, a single exception.

Were the existing mood the dominant factor in musical effect, or even a constant factor, we should expect to find such figures as those just given the characteristic ones. The percentages of those recording active effects and those recording passive effects show practically no difference in ratio except for the one number, " Blue Danube Waltz." It seems evident that the existing mood of the listener is only a minor factor. This does not mean that re-presented material, i.e. differences in the listener's temperament, his experience, his familiarity with various kinds of music, etc., are not vital factors. It does mean, however, that the music has some dominant effective quality which awakens in the listener a characteristic response. The physiological increase or decrease of energy is directly dependent upon the music and is but little influenced, except in quantity, by the already existing mood of the listener.

A study of fourteen people who described themselves as active on one evening and passive on the other showed no noticeable differences in the effect of the music. No listener recorded a dynamically different effect for Selection I and only one person failed to record on second hearing *exactly* the *same* effect that was recorded on the first hearing. This one hearer recorded *stirred* in one instance and *patriotic* in the other, both active responses. The following table shows the differences in dynamic effect which were recorded.

Selection.	Observers recording different effect on second hearing.
Stars and Stripes For Ever March	0
Menuetto All' Anti'co	3
Blue Danube Waltz	4
To a Wild Rose	0
Spring Song (Mendelssohn)	6
Anvil Chorus	1
He Shall Feed His Flock	4
Les Oiseaux dans la Charmille	0
Love's Old Sweet Song	1
Ave Maria (Bach-Gounod) (Soprano)	3

Only twenty-two cases out of the one hundred and forty show dynamically different effects on the two occasions. The response of most people is physiologically the same to a given piece of music whether they feel active or passive before listening.

A summary of the reports in answer to the question : Which selection did you like best ? Least ? shows a remarkable consistency in the rank order of the ten selections for the first and second hearings. This comparison of favourites is best shown by the following table in which the figures of column II represent the number of hearers designating each selection as *best liked*.

Selection.	First Hearing.		Second Hearing.	
	1st Choice.	Rank Order.	1st Choice.	Rank Order.
1	13	1	6	3·5
2	4	6	2	8
3	8	4	8	2
4	9	2·5	3	6
5	1	9·5	4	5
6	5	5	2	8
7	3	7	6	3·5
8	1	9·5	1	10
9	2	8	2	8
10	9	2·5	9	1

The correlation between the rank order of the ten selections on two trials is ·70. It is an interesting fact that selections 3, 5, 7 and 10 are ranked higher in the second hearing. These are musical numbers which, although not well liked at first perhaps, one comes to appreciate more and more with repeated hearings.

CONCLUSIONS

More people express a wish for music dynamically similar to the existing mood than for music of the opposite effect.

Almost the entire group shows a consistency in the relationship of the desired music to the existing mood. This means that the relation of music desired to the listener's mood is an individual difference, which relationship is fairly constant for each individual.

The music itself is the dominant factor in the effect aroused. The proportions reporting dynamic and depressing effects from a given selection are the same for the group of hearers characterizing themselves in active terms as for the group of hearers characterizing themselves in passive terms. This shows that the attitude of the listener is not as vital a factor in the effect of music upon him as is popularly supposed. Temperamental and educational differences are doubtless more important factors.

That music itself does arouse specific responses, which are constant from time to time, is evidenced by the fact that the reports of those hearers who characterized themselves as active at one hearing and as passive at the other, show only a very few variations in the dynamic effects recorded for the two times. The elements of the music itself are the most dominant factors in the effects produced.

4. *The Effect of the Induced Mood on the Subsequent Mood* [1]

We are now interested in the effect that an induced mood has on the subsequent mood. Thus, if the listener reports a certain mood as resulting from the music, does he express a preference for a continuation or for a change of that type of music, and under what conditions ? The variables that might influence the direction of the preference are the type of mood induced, and the degree of enjoyment derived from the music. On the data sheet for the study of the mood effects of music the listeners were asked to state after each selection the kind of music they would like to hear next, and if possible to name a typical selection.[2] In the majority of cases, both the kind of music preferred and the name of the composition were given. The expressed preference was then compared with the mood effect of the selection to which the person

---

[1] By Dr. Schoen.   [2] Chapter VII, p. 138.

had just listened, and a deduction made as to whether the type of music called for represented a contrast or was similar to the reported mood.

The data obtained were meagre and inconclusive, so that not much confidence can be placed in the conclusions that may be deduced from them. In the table below a summary of the data is shown :—

EFFECT OF INDUCED MOOD ON SUBSEQUENT MOOD

	Joyful-exhilarated.	Calm-restful.	Sad-depressing.
No. of Subjects Preferring Change of Mood	15	18	34
No. of Subjects Preferring Continuation of Mood . .	23	20	4

If all the moods reported as resulting from all the selections are grouped under the three general effects of (1) exhilarating, (2) restful, (3) depressing, we may conclude here in a preliminary way, that the more intense moods at the extreme ends of the mood scale, such as exhilaration and depression, arouse a desire, more or less marked, in a definite direction, the former for continuation of that type of mood and the latter for a change, while the milder moods leave the hearer in a state of indifference as to the succeeding type of music. All these effects are independent of the degree of enjoyment.

5. *Enjoyment and Mood*

The element of enjoyment is probably the one factor of greatest significance in any investigation relative to musical effects. Irrespective of the problems concerning the types of musical enjoyment, or the differences in individual attitude towards musical stimulation, or the enjoyment derived from the different elements constituting a musical composition, such as the rhythmic, melodic,

harmonic, and so forth, the mood effect must, nevertheless, be evaluated in terms of degree of enjoyment, for
the only standard available at present for judging the
intensity of emotion is in terms of its affective concomitant.

The problem presents three aspects for consideration,
(1) the relation of intensity of effect to the intensity of
pleasure, (2) the kind of mood or moods most enjoyed,
(3) kind of mood changes most enjoyed.

1. The means for determining the relationship of
mood effect to enjoyment is to compare the ranking in
pleasure of those selections having a high emotional effect
with the selections having a low emotional effect. The
data shown in the accompanying table were obtained
from the previous study on the nature of musical enjoyment.[1] Two hundred and sixty-one selections were
recorded as having high emotional effect and one hundred
and twenty-two as having low emotional effect.

TABLE SHOWING MUSICAL PLEASURE OF SELECTIONS HIGH AND
LOW IN EMOTIONAL EFFECT

Enjoyment.	Selections of High Mood Effect.	% of 261.	Selections. of Low Mood Effect.	% of 122.
Above Average.	199	76	18	15
Average . .	31	12	22	18
Below Average.	31	12	82	67
	261	100	122	100

Of the two hundred and sixty-one selections of high
emotional effect, seventy-six per cent are ranked above
average in the amount of pleasure which they gave to each
observer. On the other hand, of the one hundred and
twenty-two selections of low emotional effect, sixty-
seven per cent are ranked as below average in the amount

[1] Chapter IV, p. 86.

of pleasure. This is indicative of the fact that a high degree of pleasure is concomitant with high emotional effect, a lack of musical pleasure is accompanied by an absence of emotional effect.

Whether this emotional effect is the cause of the pleasure is another problem. It is certainly not the sole cause. The simple physiological pleasure from tones themselves is a definite form of pleasure, which may or may not be accompanied by a conscious emotional effect. The physiological reflexes stimulated by a slow-moving rhythm may give decided pleasure and yet there may be no conscious awareness of feeling or effect.

That the presence of emotional effect is correlated with the total degree of pleasure derived, is nevertheless certain. It is conceivable that the scoring on the several effects enumerated may be to some degree the same scoring as that on pleasure in another form. In other words, the scoring on the various emotions and effects may be a conscious introspective analysis of the pleasure of the selection.

The fact that the correlation between degree of pleasure and any given effect shows such consistency for several hearers, is evidence of the fact that the ratings on the affective factors are significant. Whether or not the causative relationship is accepted, it seems certain that there is a definite positive relationship between the intensity of the feeling or the emotion aroused in the hearer and the intensity of pleasure experienced.

Another means of determining the relationship of emotional effect to musical pleasure is a study of only those selections which have a high score on pleasantness. Ninety-four selections were scored high on pleasantness by each listener, and thirty others received an average score. Of the ninety-four selections reported as giving the highest degree of pleasure to all the hearers, the distribution into emotional class groups is as follows :—

Class.	Number.	%	% of Class.
I	80	85	23
II	7	7	18
III	6	7	4
IV	1	1	1

The figures of the third column indicate the relative proportions of the selections chosen for high pleasure value which fall into each of the several emotional classes. The figures in the fourth column indicate, on the other hand, the per cent of the various emotional classes which are chosen as being particularly agreeable or pleasant. These represent somewhat different angles.

The first of the two groups, namely, those selections which gave a very high degree of pleasure to each, is unquestionably the more significant. Twenty-three per cent of all the selections (Class I) which have a uniform and decided emotional effect have a very high degree of pleasure. Eighteen per cent of those selections which showed a marked emotional effect, the effect differing with each individual (Class II) rank very high in the amount of pleasure they give to each hearer. Only a very small proportion of those selections which show uniform emotional effect, but of only slight intensity (Class III), or of those selections which have no emotional effect (Class IV) give a high degree of pleasure.

From this study we also conclude, then, that a *very high* emotional feeling as a result of music is accompanied by a keen degree of enjoyment.

2 and 3. The data for the tables given below showing the relationship between degree of enjoyment and type of mood induced, and degree of enjoyment and type of mood change taking place were obtained from the

data sheet used in the study on the Mood Effects of Music.[1]

TYPE OF MOOD AND ENJOYMENTS

	Average Degree of Enjoyment.
Joyful—	
Liebesfreud	4·7
Pastel-Minuet	4·2
Anitra's Dance. . . .	4
Shepherd's Dance . . .	5
Aida March	4
Light Cavalry Overture . .	4
William Tell Overture . .	4
	—
Total Average . . .	4
Serious—	
May is Here	4
Humoresque	3
Evening Star	4
Berceuse	5
Kamennoi-Ostrow . . .	4
Ave Maria	4
Asa's Tod	5
Funeral March . . .	4
	—
Total Average . . .	4

DEGREE OF ENJOYMENT AND KIND OF MOOD CHANGE

Joyful to Serious.	Serious to Joyful.
6	6
5	5
4	6
4	6
4	6
4	5
4	3
4	6
6	6
4	4
6	5
6	5
—	—
Total Average 4	5

From the meagre data presented in these tables it appears that for the seventeen listeners used in the

[1] Chapter VII, p. 138.

experiment, the amount of enjoyment derived from musical selections resulting in a joyful mood is no greater than that derived when a serious mood is induced. The degree of enjoyment, however, as a whole, when the mood change taking place is from joyful to serious, is slightly less than that when the change is from serious to joyful.

We conclude, then, concerning the relationship between enjoyment and mood, that (1) there is a positive correlation between intensity of mood effect and enjoyment, but that (2) no greater amount of enjoyment is derived from one type of mood than from another type, unless the induced mood is due to a dislike for a specific type of music or to poor performance, and that (3) the amount of enjoyment is slightly affected by the kind of mood change taking place.

6. *Familiarity and Enjoyment*

The relationship between degree of familiarity and enjoyment is of great importance for the teaching of musical appreciation, and for the concert artist, in constructing his programmes. If there is a fixed relationship between the two factors, then it is clear that music education has here a principle to serve it as a guide in the teaching of appreciation, namely, to familiarize the pupils with the masterpieces of musical literature. Again, for the artist who still has his reputation to make with the public it would mean that he had better lay stress in his programmes upon familiar selections, and leave the novel and newer music to the artist of established reputation. The accompanying table, based on data obtained from the study on mood effects,[1] is therefore interesting from many points of view.

[1] Chapter VII, p. 138.

TABLE SHOWING RELATION OF AVERAGE DEGREE OF ENJOYMENT
TO FAMILIARITY

(the figures represent degree of enjoyment from 00, irritation, to
6, great enjoyment)

Observers.	New.	Very Familiar.	Ability to Name Selection.	Total Average for Each Listener.
W. B.	4	4	4	4
D. C.	3	–	–	–
R. D.	5	5	4	5
E. D.	3	4	4	4
E. H.	4	5	5	5
G. I.	5	6	6	6
R. K.	5	5	6	6
N. K.	4	4	4	4
L. M.	5	0	4	3
M. L.	6	–	–	–
M. M.	3	6	6	5
G. M.	6	5	4	5
P. M.	6	6	6	6
L. P.	2	3	0	2
F. R.	3	5	6	5
I. W.	3	5	4	4
	–	–	–	–
Total Average	4	6	6	4

We note here that the degree of enjoyment in the
very familiar and *ability to name* columns is, for the
great majority of the listeners, greater than in the *new*
column, and that, as a whole, the familiar selections
were enjoyed *greatly* while the *new* selections gave
moderate enjoyment. Another point worth noting,
but which calls for further investigation, is that familiarity
plays a more important rôle in the enjoyment of the
somewhat musical than in that of the markedly musical.
In other words, there is reason for believing that the less
musical the person, the more his enjoyment is conditioned
upon the degree of his familiarity with the selection.
It is further noteworthy that in the matter of degree
of enjoyment the listeners divide themselves into three
groups, namely, those whose enjoyment is both slight

and rare, those whose enjoyment is both frequent and great, those whose enjoyment is rare but great. Into the first class fall the non-musical, in the second class we find the somewhat musical, while the third class includes the most musical. The non-musical, then, as is but to be expected, enjoys music but rarely, and then but slightly, while the very musical person, whose taste is discriminating, and into whose musical judgment there enter many complex and complicating factors, particularly those relating to interpretation, likewise meets rarely with enjoyment, but when present it is intense. The very musical find themselves, then, in most cases, at either one of the two extremes, they either experience intense pleasure or very little. The somewhat musical, on the other hand, whose attitude towards music is uncritical, but who are nevertheless attracted to music, find great enjoyment most often.

7. *Effect of Enjoyment on Judgment of Quality*

What influence does enjoyment or lack of enjoyment exert upon the individual's evaluation of the quality of the music ? Does the hearer associate the two unconsciously, or are the two distinct in his mind ? The second supposition would necessarily imply that the hearer assumes a critical attitude towards his own enjoyment, pronouncing it as worthy or unworthy in terms of his evaluation of the quality of the music heard. To assume that such a process takes place sounds farfetched and unreasonable. It is rather to be expected that degree of enjoyment and judgment of quality go hand in hand, excepting in those extreme cases in which the listener is aware that he is enjoying a musical composition that is universally judged to be poor, or, in the other extreme, in which a critical attitude is deliberately assumed by the listener, an attitude that is as rare as it is probably destructive of enjoyment. Our results show that in several instances a listener reported *no enjoyment* while judging the music to be *very good*, but this apparent discrepancy is due to the fact that the lack of enjoyment was due to the rendition and not to the music itself, so that the listener was forced by conditions to separate the two items. In all other cases, judgment of quality of the music is in direct proportion to the intensity of the pleasure derived from it.

RELATION OF JUDGMENT OF SELECTION TO DEGREE
OF ENJOYMENT

	Degree of Enjoyment.				
	00	0	2	4	6
Judgment of Quality .	–	–	–	–	–
Very Good .	2	1	6	18	70
Fair . .	5	2	4	4	–
Poor. . .	2	–	–	–	–
Very Poor .	3	–	–	–	–

8. *Judgment of Selection and Familiarity*

Since we have found a close relationship between degree of enjoyment and familiarity and also between the degree of enjoyment and evaluation of musical quality the close relation between quality and familiarity, as indicated by the accompanying table, was only to be expected. Thus, we note that the *new* selections were judged to be *very good* seventeen times, while the *familiar* selections were placed in the *very good* class fifty-nine times, and of those falling into the *good* classification the *new* were mentioned nineteen times, and the *familiar* twenty-eight times. Not only is there a tendency evident to judge fewer of the *new* selections as either *very good, good,* or *fair,* but also to place most of the *familiar* selections into the *very good* class.

RELATION OF JUDGMENT OF SELECTION TO FAMILIARITY

	New.	Familiar.
Very Good . .	20	59
Good . . .	19	28
Fair . . .	6	8
Poor . . .	1	1
Very Poor . .	2	1

SECTION IV

THE ORGANIC EFFECTS OF MUSIC

Introductory Note.—The introspective methods of studying the effects of music, a procedure in which a person is called upon to analyze the mental state resulting from hearing a musical selection, is open to many objections. In the first place it is questionable whether any confidence can be placed in the report of the average person as to the subtle and complex effects of music when an analysis of even the most simple mental process requires a person trained in psychological observation. Secondly, one of the essential requirements of a sound scientific method is that the procedure be verifiable under constant conditions. The introspective method cannot meet this requirement. Thirdly, the effect that music might have upon a person when listening under normal conditions is unquestionably distorted to a considerable extent by the artificial attitude the hearer is forced into as the result of attempting an analysis of the effects of what is heard. If it is true, furthermore, as Professor Myers intimates, that self-forgetfulness, or complete absorption in the music is an important attribute of the æsthetic attitude, then the objection to the introspective method for purposes of analyzing music and its effects becomes still more serious, since the mental states in self-analysis and self-forgetfulness are certainly mutually exclusive.

That the procedure, however, is valuable, and can yield fruitful results is evident from the studies presented in the previous sections. What is needed is a check upon the introspective report of the listener in the form of the organic processes induced by the music.

The study presented in this section is of the utmost significance, in that it presents an opening wedge for such a method of procedure, and also because of the extensive data that Dr. Hyde obtained of the changes produced by contrasted musical selections on the electro-cardiograms, pulse rate, systolic, diastolic, and pulse pressure, and the rate and flow of the blood.—EDITOR.

CHAPTER IX

EFFECTS OF MUSIC UPON ELECTRO-CARDIOGRAMS AND BLOOD PRESSURE

IDA H. HYDE

A SCIENTIFIC employment of the power exerted by music for specific purposes, as for instance to lessen nervous tension or fatigue, or to arouse emotions requires not only a knowledge of the listener's preference for certain selections of music or for a special musical instrument, but it is also essential to know the psychological as well as the concomitant physiological reactions that are produced by the music. These reactions, as is well known, are the result of nerve stimuli on definite tissue cells and can be demonstrated with the aid of suitable apparatus.

The purpose of the present investigation was to ascertain the effects of different kinds of musical selections upon the cardio-vascular system in individuals who are known to be fond of music, persons indifferent or not sensitive to music, some Indian students, neurasthenics and some animals. The plan was to compare the effects of vocal music and that of different kinds of instruments upon listeners of different native endowment and training and under varying conditions, but only a beginning was made, enough, however, to prove that investigations in this field offer important returns.

The preliminary experiments were conducted on young men fond of music and under fairly constant subjective and weather conditions. From these first experiments it was learned that contrasted selections of music produced similar responses in pulse rate, pulse and blood pressure, velocity of the blood flow and action current, or electrical phenomena of the cardiac muscles. The data obtained from the selections that were familiar to the young men indicated that associated memory played a part in the results, and that the same selections produced a different effect when sung than when played on the violin. It was interesting to see that meals, certain foods, smoking, vitiated air, fatigue, familiarity and repetition, and excited and depressed states of mind all exerted an influence upon the effects produced by the music, and these varied for different individuals.

The same method that had been adopted in the preliminary investigation was employed in the continuation of the research. Of the fifteen men and women selected as listeners four were Indian students, seven were male students, two of which were not fond of music and could not distinguish one tone from another; and eight were women. Of the latter two were not sensitive to music, one was hysterical, one was an instructor in music, one had a defective heart valve, and the others were fond of music.

The items included in each record were pulse rate, systolic, diastolic, and pulse pressures, measured in millimetres of mercury, relative velocity of the blood flow, and electro-cardiograms that record the action current or electromotive force of the ventricular muscle contractions. These items were secured from one to five minutes before the music began, and from one to fifteen minutes after it had ceased. Until the persons were accustomed to the method of procedure, while listening to the music, only the cardiograms were taken, because it was found that the latter were affected by the manipulations necessary to secure the blood pressure records.

The electro-motor changes in the contraction of the cardiac muscles were obtained with an Einthoven string galvanometer. Through it, we have as is well known, for the first time a method for measuring and contrasting cardiac excitations and indirectly also changes in pulse rate and an aid in explaining changes in blood pressure.

For the comparison of musical and other stimuli the galvanometer was set for a film speed of 2·5 centimetres per second, and the time marker deflection per one millivolt. Lead " Two " was adopted for all the curves, that is, when the persons right arm and left leg are connected to the galvanometer through silver cuffs kept in place by bandages moistened with physiological salt solution.

The photographed curves of the electrical currents show the changes in excitation of the heart muscle, and afford a novel method of approach to the study of changes due to pathological, psychological, or physiological influences. Three photographs were taken on the effect of each of the musical records from each of the listeners. These photographs were compared, tabulated, and interpreted for final conclusions.

A Tycos sphygmomanometer, controlled by an Erlanger's type of the apparatus was used to get pulse rate and systolic and diastolic blood pressure. From these records the pulse pressure and the relative velocity of the blood flow were calculated. The systolic pressure was read at the onset of the first phase and the diastolic at the beginning of the fourth in every case.

The following three records that seemed to be free from associated disturbing influences were decided upon for the comparison tests for all the persons. First, the record of the Boston Symphony Orchestra of Tschaikowsky's "Symphony Pathetique" characterized by slow minor movements ; second, the Toreador's brilliant description of the bull fight, from " Carmen ", as sung by Amato ; and third the " National Emblem ", a stirring rhythmical march by Sousa's Band. On a few special cases a lullaby played on the violin was employed to test the soothing restful effects upon the cardio-vascular system.

The individuals were classified in two groups. In one were placed those that had love for and training in music, and in the other those that lacked these. When similar results were obtained from several members of the same group, the average data only were tabulated, but unusual changes were noticed and taken into consideration in the final reports.

For control data the student's records were taken without the influence of music at different hours of the day but not directly before meals or two hours after meals because it was seen that ingestion of food, its quantity and character, affects the cardio-vascular records.

It was also found that cardio-vascular changes vary somewhat during the day, and for some individuals and for certain hours more so than for others. These variations may be related to the general diurnal metabolic and physical activities of the organism and are taken into account in preparing the data. As a rule the pulse rate and relative velocity of blood flow decreased at the end of an hour's experimentation. The general results of this set of experiments agree on the whole with those published by Weysse and Lutz No. 3. The results of the experiments that were conducted in a poorly ventilated room or upon students after smoking cigarettes, or on a convalescent patient, differ in certain particulars from those obtained from normal students under normal conditions without the influence of music. With poor ventilation systolic and diastolic pressure increased and other records decreased. Smoking of long duration lowered the pulse rate and pulse pressure, and relative velocity of the blood flow. But the hour's rest while sitting for the test proved beneficial to the convalescent person whose systolic and pulse pressure and relative velocity of the blood flow all increased.

Three tests were made for each of the thirteen listeners on the influence of the orchestral music of Tschaikowsky's Symphony. Among these were included individuals of different degrees of native endowment, training, and physical conditions. The results obtained from these as demonstrated in the cardiograms vary in certain respects. Curves 60 and 62, recording the reactions from a male music student, were selected as typical for the curves of the normal listeners fond of music. Curve 60 was recorded before the symphony was heard and 62 seven minutes after it had been listened to. In comparing these curves it was seen that QR, the highest deflection and the one that records the action current of the ventricular muscle contraction covers seven scale divisions of two-tenths of a millivolt each, and equal therefore to an electromotive force of one and four-tenths millivolts, and the pulse rate had fallen to 76 per minute, a decrease of two-tenths millivolts and four heart beats per minute, due to the influence of the symphony was thus recorded. According to the statements of the listeners the minor tones of the symphony aroused depressing sensations ; these, however, were not of the same degree in all persons.

In considering therefore the information gained from a study of electro-cardiograms, together with the average results recorded for all of the normal students before the symphony was heard with the data recorded from one to seventy minutes after it had ceased, we learned that on the whole, there was a decrease in function of the cardio-vascular system excepting in the diastolic blood pressure, by the reflex stimulation of the mournful tones of the symphony.

Due to a lack of sufficient data it is not possible to state at present how long the after effects of the minor tones persist. The effects may, however, be quickly counteracted by certain selections of music that inhibit the depressed condition. This was demonstrated by presenting 15 minutes after the symphony had ceased the " National Emblem March " as played by Sousa's Band. Other cheering stimuli may have the same effect. On the other hand, the listener is placed by the minor tones in a receptive or susceptible mood for stimuli of a discouraging or depressing character.

For the purpose of testing the effect of the symphony on a convalescent person responses were secured from a hysterical patient. Cardiograms were taken before, and one minute after, and also ten minutes after the convalescent had listened to the music. It was apparent that the minor tones affected and distressed her. Within a minute after hearing the symphony her systolic pressure rose from 112 to 118 mm. Hg., diastolic from 68 to 80, pulse rate from 78 to 90 per minute, but E.M.F. fell from 0·8 to 0·65 and the pulse pressure from 44 to 38. But ten minutes later the patient seemed faint and it was surprising to see that the records were reversed, showing a fall below those obtained before the music was heard.

Another interesting experiment was the influence of

the symphony on the instructor in music, fatigued after a day's teaching.   After listening to the music she remarked that she disliked it.   The curves and data showed that five minutes after the music ceased the cardio-vascular records excepting the pulse pressure and E.M.F. of the heart muscle increased and then fell.   In both of the last two types of individuals there was, after hearing the music a marked rise of all the cardio-vascular functions excepting the pulse pressure and E.M.F. of the heart muscle.   This was followed ten minutes later by a remarkable reversed action of the cardio-vascular activities, which in the case of the convalescent was a change to less than what they were before the symphony had been heard.

As a result of these experiments it is safe to say, that music of the character of the symphony is not to be recommended for individuals who are fatigued, depressed, or ill.   It might be employed to subdue hilarity in individuals or masses of people.

The average results of the influences of the symphony on persons neither fond of nor sensitive to music were next tabulated and electro-cardiograms obtained before the symphony had been heard and after it had been repeated several times.   In comparing the cardiograms and data furnished by this set of students, it was seen that the results obtained before they listened to the music with those secured after they had heard it were practically alike, and very different from those of Group A.   Evidently for the persons that lacked sympathy for music the minor symphony tones neither inhibited nor stimulated the nervous control of the functions of the cardio-vascular system under consideration, nor the emotions of depression or sadness.

The influence of Toreador's song from " Carmen ",

describing the bull fight was next investigated. The cardiograms recorded from the listeners that were fond of and sensitive to music demonstrated that the song did not have the same physiological or psychological effect on all of the listeners. In those persons that had enjoyed the song very much, all of the reactions excepting that of the diastolic blood pressure were augmented. But three of the listeners did not enjoy the song, and their reactions were not increased but more or less lowered. The Indian student remarked that there was a challenge in the spirit of the song that annoyed him. It was found that his reaction had not become greater. The instructor of music was familiar with the song, had very often heard it and did not especially care for it. In her case the results showed that the effect of familiarity and repetition of music that was indifferent had little or no effect on the cardio-vascular system. The song disturbed a listener who was in poor health, but a month later when she was quite well she enjoyed the song and the reactions due to it were then reversed, that is increased. A study of the cardiograms and records secured from persons not fond of or sensitive to music showed that the Toreador's song exerted neither a psychological nor a physiological influence on these persons. As a result of these experiments we may conclude that the brilliant tones of the Toreador's song stimulated the cardio-vascular functions to increased activity in those individuals that found pleasure in the song. On the other hand, it did not augment the functions in those that did not enjoy it. Moreover, the song exerted no influence on the persons that are not fond of music. It is not known from these experiments whether it was the spirit inherent in the song or the musical and vocal tones that produced the greater effect.

We shall now consider the influences of the rhythmical "National Emblem" played by Sousa's Band. On all of the sensitive listeners excepting on the music teacher, that did not care for this sort of music, the rhythmical band music had a stimulating effect, and proved enjoyable. Moreover, it was especially the systolic and pulse pressures and relative velocity of the blood flow that were stimulated to increased activity by the stirring tones. It was interesting to see how quickly this music had a bracing effect and removed fatigue. Then, too, the depressed responses to the minor tones of the tragic symphony were counteracted and again restored to their normal activities by the rhythmical sounds of this gay composition rendered by the musical instruments. On two of the non-sensitive listeners who recognized a difference between this and the other selections, this march produced a slight and increased reaction. But neither the stolid Indian girl nor the man who could not keep step seemed to be affected by even this class of music or instruments.

It finally became of interest to ascertain the effects of an Indian war song that was whooped and sung by the composer of the song to the drum accompaniment. The listeners were unprepared for this performance. It was not surprising therefore that the weird war tones and beating of the drum affected each of the listeners differently. On a male music student much interested in the composition of sounds it first produced a great rise in systolic and pulse pressure, 106 to 114 and 56 to 62 respectively, but a fall in all of the other reactions for about fifteen minutes' duration, during which the pulse had fallen from 84 to 75 per minute. But in a convalescent, the tremendous effect was at once a marked decrease, especially of the systolic pressure 110 to 98, and velocity of the blood flow that lasted more than thirteen minutes.

Judging from impressions and records obtained during and after the performances the effect on her was more like a shock. Also on a woman fond of music who had never heard anything of the kind, the sounds produced a shock-like effect resulting in a fall of all of the cardio-vascular activities, excepting that a most remarkable increase in the electromotive force of the cardiac muscles took place.

On the other hand, on an Indian man fond of music and familiar with Indian songs, the sounds produced surprise and pleasure. His records during the time of the performance showed an increase in 10 beats in pulse rate, 6 mm. in diastolic blood pressure and 0·2 millivolts in electromotive force, thus showing a striking difference in results from those above noted. The performance had some effect on an instructor in music who had often heard the song and was always amused by it. Here, then, was a type of music that actually had a psychological and physiological effect on the non-sensitive Indian listeners. As soon as the wild war song and sounds of the drum fell upon their ears the man, belonging to an Indian football team, was agreeably surprised. All his records excepting the pulse rate greatly increased during the rendering of the song and for at least eight minutes afterward. It seemed, however, that the unexpected performance suddenly robbed the Indian woman of her stolidity and left her in a sort of dazed condition. Her reactions excepting the diastolic pressure fell at once and remained below normal for about eight minutes. It may be said, however, that on the whole more often as a first result, the rendering of this selection produced a depression of the cardio-vascular activities on those listeners who had been unaccustomed to this kind of performance or for whom it recalled emotional associations, or who found it distressing. On the other hand, for those Indian listeners who enjoyed it and for whom the surprise was not powerful enough to counteract the pleasure of the song, the reactions of the cardio-vascular system under discussion were increased. The effect of this wild war song may be likened to a reflex shock produced by strong stimulations. The after effect or emotional durability varied for the different individuals.

Another experiment was undertaken to test the effect of a lullaby played on a violin, upon a woman patient who appeared to suffer from nutritional disturbances as a consequence of influenza. The electro-cardiac records, however, revealed a disorder of the heart's action ; an extreme auricular acceleration, or auricular flutter. The auricular contractions were conspicuously displayed by the shadow of the needle on the camera, and the influence of the lullaby on the patient distinctly observed in all its details. Both her husband and the experimenter were amazed at the suddenness of the change in the cardiac contractions when the lullaby was heard. In some of the tests the deflections of the flutter decreased, in others they apparently ceased. The systolic and pulse pressure and relative velocity of the blood flow were increased, but the pulse rate and the electromotive force of the ventricular muscle decreased. The musical tones proved restful and beneficial to the patient. From the conspicuously beneficial effects produced upon the activities of the heart and the tonicity of the cardio-vascular system in general it is safe to recommend the lullaby as a sedative influence for individuals who are sensitive to musical tones.

The selections employed in this investigation may not be considered ideal ones for testing the effects of music upon individuals whose native musical endowment and training are very different. Nevertheless it has been demonstrated through their use that certain selections of music and most likely certain musical instruments and qualities of the vocal sounds exert a far-reaching influence upon the cardio-vascular system and very likely upon other functions of the body. It is probable that the employment of certain selections of music will prove a valuable aid in the treatment of nervous disorders.

SUMMARY

It has been discovered that cardio-vascular functions are reflexly stimulated concomitantly with psychological effects of music and that, through the use of the Einthoven string galvanometer, and sensitive sphygmomanometers, the physiological reactions that have been excited by different sorts of music can be measured and compared.

Moreover, with this method the proper sort of music may be prescribed and thus a scientific employment of the power inherent in music may prove a valuable adjunct to psychotherapy in the treatment of convalescent or other patients sensitive to music.

On persons not susceptible to music the tragic minor tones that characterized Tschaikowsky's symphony were without effect. But in persons endowed with musical sensitivity the tones of the selections produced a stimulation that as a rule reflexly lowered the functions especially considered in this investigation. This class of music is therefore not to be recommended for individuals depressed, fatigued, or convalescent, but may be employed to subdue hilarity. The general effect of the Toreador's song was an increase in the functions of the cardio-vascular system. The results varied with the individual and depended upon the health, native endowment, musical training, also upon the interpretation of the theme and familiarity with the selection, and moreover upon the degree to which it was enjoyed or disliked. The song exerted no influence upon those listeners that were not sensitive to music or those that were familiar with the song but did not care for it.

As a rule, the records secured on the effect of the "National Emblem March", showed an increase in the cardio-vascular activity, especially noticeable in the velocity of the blood flow and systolic and diastolic blood pressure. But for those who were not able to keep step with the march and lacked fondness for music the records remained unchanged. This sort of music proved valuable in counteracting depressed reactions produced by the minor tones of the symphony, in removing fatigue, and arousing muscular activity.

The song of the Indian war dance accompanied by the drum was the only music that exerted an influence upon the stolid non-sensitive Indian listeners. The Indian man was agreeably surprised by the performance. His records rose far above his normal ones. The Indian woman, however, was bewildered by the unexpected thrilling sounds and all of her reactions, excepting the diastolic blood pressure, were greatly decreased. The psychological and concomitant physiological reactions, excited partly by surprise and partly by the startling barbaric combination of tones varied for the different sensitive listeners.

From the conspicuously beneficial results exerted upon the activities of the heart, inhibiting auricular flutter in a patient and increasing the cardio-vascular tonicity in general, it is safe to recommend a lullaby played on the violin as a sedative for all individuals who are sensitive to musical tones.

We may conclude from the results of this investigation that most people are unfavourably affected psychologically and physiologically by music that is characterized by tragic mournful tones, and favourably affected by gay rhythmical rich toned harmonic melodies. Individual differences in native endowment and training are accompanied by individual differences in physiological reactions to certain musical compositions.

The indications are, that those selections of music rendered either vocally or instrumentally that exert a favourable reflex-action on the cardio-vascular system, have also a favourable influence upon the muscle tone, working power, digestion, secretions, and other functions of the body.

Vocal and instrumental music may be selected that will excite psychological and concomitant cardio-vascular reactions the effect of which might inhibit irritability, act as a sedative, arouse optimism, and be used as a valuable agent to scientifically organized labour.

SECTION V

THE EFFECTS OF REPETITION AND FAMILIARITY

Introductory Note. — The battle between the so-called classical and popular tastes in music is raging more intensely to-day than ever before, irritated probably by the advent and the conquest of jazz. It is quite evident that if the battle is ever to be settled at all satisfactorily it will be only though the intervention of scientific experimentation.

John Ruskin draws two distinctions in art, the first between real art and sham art, and the second between real art that is great and something else that is real art but not great. Philosophers, psychologists, and æstheticians have been attempting for centuries to find a criterion, or criteria, for such a distinction between grades of æsthetic values.

For this problem, the studies presented in this section are very illuminating, since all of them point to at least one criterion on the basis of which musical selections may be classified as to value. Two of the studies centre about the relatively lasting qualities of various kinds of music, from the most widely popular to the most severely classical. Professor Washburn and her collaborators find that when compositions of various types are played and immediately repeated several times, the result of the repetitions is that the degree of pleasure and interest wanes more rapidly for the popular selections than for the classical, the exact degree and intensity of the waning interest and pleasure depending upon the musicalness of the hearer. Professors Gilliland and Moore confirm these conclusions and also find like results when selections of different types are repeated after considerable intervals of time. Professor Downey and her collaborator give the results of a study made on the result of repetition, namely, familiarity, on the sequence of numbers in a musical programme.

Again it is noteworthy that the three independent studies are strikingly uniform in the conclusions reached. —EDITOR.

CHAPTER X

THE EFFECT OF IMMEDIATE REPETITION ON THE PLEASANT-
NESS OR UNPLEASANTNESS OF MUSIC

Margaret Floy Washburn, Margaret S. Child, and
Theodora Mead Abel

THE effect of repetition on the agreeableness or dis-
agreeableness of music under ordinary circumstances
is usually that exerted by repetitions with a considerable
time interval between them. We hear the same piece
of music performed on different occasions intermittently,
we do not hear it repeated again and again on the same
occasion. The conditions under which the experimenters
in this study had to work made it highly inconvenient,
however, to secure reports from a large number of
observers who came on a number of successive occasions.
Therefore, the problem here investigated is that of the
effect of immediate repetition rather than that of
distributed repetitions. Its exact nature will be clear
in the next section.

A section of a phonograph record was played;
after an interval of thirty seconds, allowing time for
resetting, it was repeated. This procedure was continued
until five performances of the section had been given.
Then, after an interval of two minutes, another section,
of a different record, was similarly treated. Eight
records were used in an experiment. The sections were
always the first part of the records, and so chosen as to
occupy about one minute in playing. They were always
long enough to allow for the completion of a theme,
and thus possessed musical completeness.

The listeners were in groups, ranging in size from two to twenty-four persons on different occasions of the performance of the experiment. It was explained to each group at the beginning of the sitting that the object of the experiment was to observe what changes in their attitude towards a selection would occur as it was repeated five times. Each person was provided with a sheet ruled so as to have eight vertical columns corresponding to the eight records used in an experiment, and five horizontal rows corresponding to the five repetitions given to each record. The observers were instructed, at the beginning of an experimental sitting, to record in the proper square the degree of pleasantness experienced at each repetition of a record, using a scale of five, one being the lowest degree and five the highest degree of pleasantness. They were also told to record any comments that occurred to them regarding reasons for the change in affective value, the presence of imagery or emotional content, or anything else that seemed relevant. They were requested to abstract as far as possible from outside disturbances, from the medium of the performance, from noises connected with the phonograph ; from everything, in short, except the music itself. They were also instructed not to compare judgments with their neighbours.

To counteract the effect of the time sequence of the compositions, involving that of affective contrast, in half of the experimental settings made with a given set of records, the order in time of the records was the reverse of that followed in the other half of the experimental sittings.

The experimenter, who was responsible for starting and stopping the phonograph and for changing the records, stood during the playing with her face turned away from the group of observers, in order not to serve as a source of disturbance and suggestions.

In the course of the investigation, two sets of records were used, which will be called Set I and Set II. The plan of selection followed in both sets was the same, and the two sets were intended to be similar in character. Each set included four types of records, as follows: severely classical, serious popular classical, easy popular classical, popular. The selection was made with the advice of a member of the music department, a musical expert of some distinction and an authority on the history and theory of music. The attempt was made to have the selections as unfamiliar as possible; where they were recognized, the observers were to record the fact.

For the sake of uniformity, it was planned to use only orchestral selections. Owing to the difficulty of finding enough orchestral records which met the other demands of the experiment, three violin records were introduced, two in Set I and one in Set II.

In the case of each of the four types of records in a set, one record of slow tempo and one of quick tempo was included.

The records used were the following :—

	Set.	Fast.	Slow.
Severely classical	I.	Schubert : First movement from the Unfinished Symphony (B minor).	Mozart : Quartet in D major, Andante.
	II.	Beethoven : Quartet in C major, Fugue.	Wagner : Træume.
Serious popular classical	I.	Tschaikowsky : Scherzo in E flat minor.	Schubert : Minuet in A minor.
	II.	Haydn : Military Symphony, Allegro.	Haydn : Surprise Symphony, Andante cantabile e vivace.
Easy popular classical .	I.	Wolf-Ferrari : Intermezzo from Jewels of the Madonna.	Tschaikowsky : Adante cantabile from String Quartet.
	II.	Nicolai : Merry Wives of Windsor : Overture	Mendelssohn : On Wings of Song (Heifetz).
Popular . . .	I.	Kismet Fox Trot	On Miami's Shore, Waltz.
	II.	Sultan One Step.	Rosalie Waltz.

The total number of persons with whom Set I was used was   .   117
The total number of persons with whom Set II was used was   .   103
The entire number of persons was thus   220

All of the listeners were young women college students. The attempt was made to divide them into a musically gifted and trained and a musically untrained and ungifted group, according to the answers to the following questionary :—

I.   Have you ever had music lessons ?   How long ?   Did you enjoy them ?

II.   If you have had music lessons, did you have difficulty in keeping time accurately ?

III.   Can you carry a tune ?

IV.   Have you ever studied harmony or musical theory ?   How long ? Did you enjoy it ?

V.   Have you difficulty in keeping step when dancing ?   Does it irritate you to be out of step when walking with anyone ?

VI.   Is your family musical ?

VII.   When you hear music can you tell whether or not it is in tune ?

In addition to the questionary answers, the experimenter's personal knowledge of the listeners was used as evidence in a number of cases. It is probable, however, that the division into musical and unmusical groups was not very accurate.

The number of observers classed as musical was 107.
The number of observers classed as unmusical was 113.

1.   *The Changes in Pleasantness of the Selections on Repetition*

To show these changes, the following treatment of the results was used, as being better adapted to give full value to individual variations, which were naturally very considerable in degree, than the presentation of averages of the numerical values assigned to degrees of pleasantness.   For each selection the number of cases was counted where the degree of pleasantness at the fifth performance was reported by a listener to be greater than the degree of pleasantness at the first performance. These were called *plus* cases.   The number of cases was counted where a listener had found the selection in question less agreeable on the fifth than at the first presentation ; these were called *minus* cases. For each selection, the number of *plus* cases was divided by the number of *minus* cases. This gave a series of ratios whose value was greater in proportion as repetition tended to increase the pleasantness of a selection, and less in proportion as repetition tended to diminish its pleasantness. For it should be noted that our method of studying the effect of immediate repetitions rather than that of widely distributed repetitions had this advantage, that the variations in the degree of pleasantness assigned to a selection might, in the case of repetitions separated by hours or days, be due to a great variety of causes, producing variations in the observer's affective state, while variations in pleasantness when repetitions are separated only by thirty seconds' interval must be due mainly to the repetition itself.

The ratios obtained were as follows :—

GROUP I.

Observers.	Compositions.							
	1	2	3	4	5	6	7	8
Musical . .								
(number : 54)	1·9	1·46	1·10	·93	·94	2·41	·47	·31
Unmusical								
(number : 63)	·80	1·1	·82	2·00	1·36	1·22	·69	·28

GROUP II.

Observers.	Compositions.							
	1	2	3	4	5	6	7	8
Musical . .								
(number : 53)	1·33	1·38	1·00	·65	·94	1·5	·58	·39
Unmusical .								
(number : 50)	1·72	1·11	1·06	1·63	1·53	·86	·76	·57

From this table two inferences may be drawn :—

(1) Repetition may operate either to raise or to lower the pleasantness of a selection.

(2) In the case of popular music repetition tends more strongly to lower than to raise pleasantness.

(Obviously, since the ratios are obtained by dividing the number of persons who found a selection more agreeable on the fifth than on the first presentation by the number who found it less agreeable on the fifth than on the first presentation, where a ratio is close to unity the tendencies to raise and to lower pleasantness on repetition were about equal in amount : where a ratio exceeds unity, there is a greater tendency to raise than to lower, and where a ratio falls below unity there is a greater tendency to lower than to raise.)

(3) Except in the case of very popular music, five immediate repetitions have a somewhat greater tendency to raise than to lower the pleasantness of a selection. There are sixteen ratios above unity to seven below unity.

We also recorded for each person and each composition the repetition at which the composition reached its highest degree of pleasantness. By adding we found for each composition and each repetition the number of observers who had experienced the greatest degree of pleasantness at that repetition. The following table shows the results :—

GROUP I

Musical Observers.   Compositions.

		1	2	3	4	5	6	7	8
Performance	1 .	12	17	17	18	13	13	(20)	(32)
,,	2 .	15	19	(23)	21	25	12	17	21
,,	3 .	18	25	17	(23)	(26)	14	16	15
,,	4 .	(19)	24	16	22	20	(28)	11	8
,,	5 .	18	(26)	21	20	15	(28)	12	6

Unmusical Observers.

		1	2	3	4	5	6	7	8
Performance	1 .	18	20	19	16	21	15	(24)	(26)
,,	2 .	23	(27)	12	18	26	19	19	21
,,	3 .	22	21	18	23	18	21	15	15
,,	4 .	(31)	25	13	(30)	19	16	15	13
,,	5 .	29	(27)	(22)	(30)	(27)	(28)	17	13

GROUP II

Musical Observers.			Compositions.						
		1	2	3	4	5	6	7	8
Performance 1 .		17	17	(21)	20	16	11	(20)	(23)
,, 2 .		22	16	(21)	(23)	20	16	15	20
,, 3 .		22	16	(21)	16	(30)	(19)	15	21
,, 4 .		23	20	18	13	19	18	10	14
,, 5 .		(34)	(21)	18	15	19	(19)	13	8

Unmusical Observers.									
Performance 1 .		14	20	17	16	15	17	(20)	(20)
,, 2 .		17	17	19	10	16	(23)	16	16
,, 3 .		19	16	(22)	15	19	18	10	17
,, 4 .		17	18	19	13	20	11	13	12
,, 5 .		(21)	(21)	18	(24)	(21)	17	12	13

It should be noted that whenever a listener reported the maximum pleasantness at two different performances of a selection, for instance, the first and third, a maximum was credited to both performances. This explains why the columns in the foregoing table do not add up to the same totals.

From the table it may be inferred that :—

(1) In the case of the very popular selections (7 and 8), the tendency is to reach the maximum at an early performance ; in the case of the seriously classical compositions (1 and 2), the tendency is to reach the maximum at a late performance. Thus, the conditions which decrease pleasantness through repetition are more operative for extremely popular music : those which increase it are more operative for seriously classical music.

(2) The tendency to lose pleasantness on repetition sets in on the whole sooner for the musical than for the unmusical observers. This is not noticeable in the seriously classical compositions at all : it is shown in the very popular selections only by a steeper dropping off of the number from the first to the fifth performance ; it appears clearly in every composition of the other two

groups (3 and 6 inclusive) with the exception of composition 6 in Group II, where the musical observers tend to reach a maximum pleasure later than the unmusical observers. The figures suggest the conclusion that musical observers are sooner satiated by immediate repetitions of a composition than unmusical observers are, except in the case of seriously classical compositions, where the reverse is the case. With regard to the exception constituted by composition 6 of Group II, the fact is probably not without significance that this composition was by both musical and unmusical groups assigned the highest degree of pleasantness of any composition in either group. This point will be discussed below.

2. *Influences Causing Change in the Degree of Pleasantness on Repetition.*

Fatigue is the influence universally reported by our listeners' introspections as causing a drop in the pleasantness of a selection on repetition. On the other hand, the influences introspectively reported as causing a rise in pleasantness are varied. The most frequently alleged reason accompanying increased pleasantness is the occurrence of *agreeable imagery*. It was mentioned by both musical and unmusical persons in 25 per cent of the introspective comments on rise of pleasantness : more accurately, in 27·9 per cent in the case of the unmusical persons and 29·3 per cent in the case of the musical persons.

For the musical persons, the other influences mentioned were as follows :—

Increased comprehension of the composition, 13·8%.
Greater attention to melody, 12·3%.
Increased familiarity, 9·3%.
Greater attention to rhythm, 9·3%.

"Getting used to it" (where original pleasantness was low:
  affective adaptation), 6·1%.
Better adjustment of mood to that of composition, 6·1%.
Greater attention to harmony, 4·6%.
Associations, 3%.

For the unmusical persons, the other influences mentioned were as follows :—

Greater attention to rhythm, 15·1%.
Increased familiarity, 13·8%.
Increased comprehension of the composition, 11·6%.
"Getting used to it," 11·6%.
Increased attention to melody, 6·9%.
"Improves with hearing" (no explanation), 4·6%.
Better adjustment to mood, 3·4%.
Associations, 2·3%.
Greater attention to piano, 2·3%.

The points of possible significance, in comparing musical and unmusical persons are that the musical persons pay more attention to comprehension of the composition, to melody, to harmony and instrumentation, and to adjustment of mood than do the unmusical persons. The latter pay more attention to familiarity, to rhythm, and to affective adaptations.

An influence revealed not by introspective reports but by consideration of the numerical returns is that of the original pleasantness of the composition. There is some tendency to find that a composition increases in pleasantness more the greater the degree of its pleasantness at the outset. This tendency would no doubt appear more clearly if it were not for the obvious fact that when the first hearing of a composition results in grade 5 of pleasantness, the listeners probably do not feel at liberty to go above 5 in expressing the pleasantness of subsequent performances.

The evidence that the pleasanter compositions wear better than the less pleasant compositions is as follows :—

For each of the four sets of persons mentioned on pages 204, 205 (Group I, Musical, Group I, Unmusical, Group II, Musical, Group II, Unmusical), the eight compositions were arranged in the order of the size of the ratios given on page 203 : the order, that is, of their tendency to increase in pleasantness on repetition. The average degree of pleasantness assigned to each composition by the observers in the given group was then found, and the eight compositions were arranged in the order of their initial pleasantness. The following rank difference correlations were then found between the two arrays :—

> Group I. Musical : Plus ·53, P.E. ·176
> ,,   I. Unmusical : Plus ·75, P.E. ·105
> ,,   II. Musical : Plus ·48, P.E. ·195
> ,,   II. Unmusical : Minus ·26, P.E. ·23

In order to secure a longer array, the following procedure was adopted. It will be remembered that to avoid a succession error, in half the experiments with a group of compositions they were presented in the order : Classical to Popular, and in the other half, in the order : Popular to Classical. The values used in the above correlations were calculated separately for the *Straight* and *Reversed* divisions of each musical and each unmusical group. Thus, sixty-four ranks were obtained. The coefficient obtained from these was plus ·35, P.E. ·077. When the thirty-two musical groups were separated from the thirty-two unmusical groups, and separate correlations found for musical and unmusical, the coefficients were as follows :

> Musical : Plus ·51, P.E. ·13
> Unmusical : Plus ·12, P.E. ·17

These figures would seem to indicate that there is some tendency for more pleasant compositions to wear better than less pleasant compositions, and that this tendency is more marked in the case of the musical persons. For this latter fact no explanation is suggested by any of our results. It will be recalled that the only exception to the rule that the musical listeners, for all except the most seriously classical compositions, tended to reach the maximum enjoyment at an earlier repetition than did the unmusical listeners, occurred in the case of composition 6 of Group II, and that this composition was the one whose initial pleasantness stood highest of all the compositions in both Group I and Group II. Its extreme initial pleasantness, together with the tendency of the musical persons to continue enjoyment of compositions longer the greater their initial pleasantness, may explain the occurrence of this exception.

SUMMARY OF RESULTS

For young women college students, five immediately consecutive performances on the phonograph of orchestral selections about one minute long, and ranging through four grades from seriously classical to very popular (both inclusive), produce influences tending to raise and influences tending to lower the pleasantness of the selection.

In the case of very popular music, the influences tending to lower pleasantness are more marked than those tending to raise it.

The tendency to lose pleasantness on repetition sets in on the whole sooner for musical than for non-musical observers, if the two groups are separated according to their answers to the questionary on page 202.

Introspections report fatigue to be the cause of diminished pleasantness on repetition.

P

The causes of increased pleasantness on repetition are : agreeable imagery, increased comprehension of the composition, increased familiarity, greater attention to rhythm, greater attention to melody, greater attention to instrumentation, greater attention to harmony, better adjustment of observer's mood to that of the composition " getting used to " the more unpleasant compositions, that is, affective adaptation ; " associations ", greater attention to piano.

Of these sources, better comprehension of the composition, greater attention to melody, to harmony, and to instrumentation, and better adjustment of mood were mentioned by more musical than unmusical observers : increased familiarity, greater attention to rhythm, and " getting used to it " were mentioned by more unmusical than musical observers.

These sources of increased pleasantness explain why simple popular music tended to decrease rather than to increase in pleasantness with repetition. Nearly all of them are influences which require complexity, in order that attention may turn from one feature to another of the composition.

Especially for musical persons, the pleasanter compositions tend to increase in pleasantness on repetition more than do the less pleasant compositions.

CHAPTER XI

THE IMMEDIATE AND LONG-TIME EFFECTS OF CLASSICAL AND POPULAR PHONOGRAPH SELECTIONS

A. R. Gilliland and H. T. Moore

AN important issue before the musical public to-day is that of classical versus popular music. In the public schools, where the phonograph has become a recognized part of educational equipment ; in the home, where some form of musical activity is coming to be the almost invariable rule ; and even in the concert hall, the battle of classicism and jazz, like that of good and evil, is being fought daily. Extreme supporters of one tendency or the other tend to range themselves in opposing camps, and the fight is waged on the one hand with the moral purpose of ridding culture of an alleged curse of degeneracy, and on the other with the cheerful determination to make clear the meaning of freedom in a democratic society.

The moral implications that have been read into this æsthetic controversy have produced more heat than light. As long as it remains a question of personal prejudice we shall never have a clear or a satisfactory solution. It remains for experimental psychology to make its contribution toward the solution of the problem by an analysis of some of the more important factors, and by an impartial statement of any general tendencies which are to be attributed to either type of music. Here is a large, important and practically unexplored territory, inviting scientific psychology to attempt the conquest.

The experiment here reported was suggested by the

commonly observed fact that a piece of so-called " jazz " music ordinarily has a more immediate appeal to a mind that is musically undeveloped than does a piece of the sort that would be played at a symphony concert. Not only is this true, but experience seems to show that attempts at direct suppression of jazz interest are likely to have an abortive result. The unconscious trends that operate in favour of street music seem to struggle for expression. Supervisors of public school music testify that the child who has had pure music artificially forced on him will, on leaving school, at once revert to the cheaper music that he has had to suppress. But the testimony of these same supervisors is unanimous that while children cannot be driven away from cheap music they can be lured away from it, if only their interest in good music is developed along natural lines. Nothing is deader than a last year's popular fox-trot, and nothing more vitally interesting than a favourite classic for one who enjoys good music.

Our problem was to make a quantitative comparison of certain effects of classical and jazz music after the first and twenty-fifth hearings. We made use of four phonograph selections. The two representing classical music were a record of Beethoven's Fifth Symphony, First Movement, and one of Tschaikowsky's Sixth Symphony, the " Pathetique ", First Movement. The two selections representing popular or jazz music were a fox-trot, entitled " That's It—A Fox-trot ", and a one-step, entitled " Umbrellas to Mend ". Each trial consisted of five hearings of each of the four records and the complete experiment consisted of five trials, or twenty-five hearings. Thirty-five of the fifty-four subjects who began the experiment were able to be present at every trial.

The effect of the music was recorded in five ways :

1.   A judgment of the enjoyment value of the piece, recorded as an estimate on a scale of ten points.

2.   A record of the speed of tapping in a thirty-second trial before and after the hearing of the music.

3.   A record of strength of grip before and after the music.

4.   A record of the pulse beat under ordinary conditions and during the music.

5.   A photograph showing the facial expression while the music was being heard.

The initial familiarity of the two types of music was practically the same, as only 3 of the subjects remembered ever having heard either of the two classical pieces, and only 4 of them felt that there was anything familiar about either of the two jazz selections.

The accompanying table gives the complete data for each of the thirty-five subjects for the first and last effects of the four selections.   The records are tabulated in the order that the pieces were always heard, namely, Beethoven, Tschaikowsky, fox-trot, one-step.   The first four columns following the initials of the subject give his records after the first hearing.   The last four columns give the corresponding records after the twenty-fifth hearing. Column 1 gives the enjoyment value of a piece after the first hearing ; column 5 gives the enjoyment value after the last hearing.   Column 2 gives the tapping record immediately after the first hearing ; column 6 the corresponding record after the last hearing   Similarly, columns 3 and 7 give the first and last records of strength of grip ; and columns 4 and 8 the first and last records of the pulse.   The photographs following the tables give the first and last facial expressions of the subjects for both the classical and the jazz music.

TABLE I

Name	First Records				Last Records			
	Rank	Tapping	Grip	Pulse	Rank	Tapping	Grip	Pulse
W. A.	8	206	52		9	224	64	68
	6	205	60½		8	216	56	70
	1	219	59½		7	205	61	68
	5	217	58		5	212	60	70
E. B.	5	163	43	80	8	195	46	75
	6	178	40½	78	7	202	51	68
	8	178	42½	83	4	195	48	70
	4	163	44	82	4	202	46½	72
H. C.	5	234	52½	92	5	241	56	95
	4	244	47½	90	4	234	58	96
	5	226	50	91	7	220	58	100
	5	245	49½	85	6	239	58	97
R. L.	7	182		84	9	184	54	75
	1	187		81	7	185	54	76
	5	189		87	4	167	51	78
	5	191		84	5	175	50	78
J. L.	6		55	87		190	43	75
	7		42	88		200	44½	77
	0		44	92		206	44½	78
	0		47	90		213	43½	78
L. M.	5	191	50	91	6	194	52	96
	6	185	50	93	5	184	53	94
	6	199	51	95	7	200	51	96
	7	176	50½	97	7	196	50	93
C. T.	7	197	43½	71	8	190	45	81
	3	192	45½	76	9	182	47	79
	4	193	46	75	5	185	45	81
	4	183	41	77	7	188	40	80
E. T.	6	214	54	66	9	234	50½	78
	6	217	50	63	10	230	49½	76
	6	222	53½	66	0	212	47	82
	1	223	53½	67	0	217	48	80
N. A.	3	216	54	75	3	236	59½	63
	2	206	49½	76	4	240	60	60
	3	228	53	84	4	234	61½	60
	4	225	54	81	3	279	59	60
C. W.	6	187	53	77	3	186	53½	72
	5	200	58	70	8	188	62	66
	6	186	52½	77	9	182	56	69
	4	188	49	78	4	184	56½	67

TABLE I (continued)

Name	First Records				Last Records			
	Rank	Tapping	Grip	Pulse	Rank	Tapping	Grip	Pulse
J. W.	7	173	48½	74	8	167	61	76
	3	156	50	73	7	166	58	74
	6	162	57	76	3	165	59½	76
	2	161	56	74	0	168	60	78
R. S.	3	284	47	77	3	319	48	94
	7	297	46½	74	5	303	54	90
	3	264	48½	79	5	331	50½	96
	2	241	45½	79	4	313	55	90
R. W.	6	189	62	80	5	207	60½	62
	6	196	58½	78	6	206	60½	63
	6	198	57	81	5	211	56	64
	4	177	58	79	4	208	56	68
C. G.	6½	281	58	83	8½	271	57½	92
	8½	270	55	89	9½	265	60	85
	8	272	55	92	4	272	56	92
	9	275	54	84	3	272	56	98
W. G.	8	194	46	87	6½	204	50½	91
	7	198	48	85	6	207	56½	93
	5	202	43	89	3	204	61	96
	4	197	45	85	3	195	53	93
J. H.	4	228	51	72	4	224	49½	64
	5	232	47	69	5	238	52	64
	4	240	55	74	5	224	51	69
	6	250	53	74	4	236	50	68
J. A.	5	235			8	235	77½	51
	7	249			7	242	76½	48
	2	243			4	234	75	53
	3	237			3	251	75	54
A. C.	7	177	52	72	5	239	65	69
	8	180	66	71	5	244	62	65
	5	220	68	72	7	226	62	64
	5	211	70	76	6	233	62	64
W. D.	5	215	52	75	7	220	54½	62
	7	230	47	75	8	220	55	64
	3	227	53	76	4	199	55½	74
	2	226	53	82	4	219	55½	73
F. D.	5	177	52	67	7	181	50½	64
	4	178	57	71	5	178	57	64
	3	181	57	73	5	170	53	64
	3	180	57	70	4	172	56	64

TABLE I (*continued*)

Name	First Records				Last Records			
	Rank	Tap-ping	Grip	Pulse	Rank	Tap-ping	Grip	Pulse
J. G.	4	193	64½	68	4	194	63½	64
	6	192	68	76	6	193	60	61
	5	209	66½	81	3	197	67	62
	5	212	66	79	5	193	66	63
W. K.	4	185	63	68	7	178	67	60
	3	179	58	67	9	184	68½	61
	2	169	64	70	2	182	69	63
	2	177	68	68	1	176	68½	62
E. L.	6		58½	58	4	195	58½	62
	3		59	61	7	210	58	64
	1		58	61	4	210	62	64
	6		55	61	5	208	59	62
L. N.	8	217	54	71	7	252	57	89
	7	227	62	70	9	242	57	89
	5	227	57	68	6	239	56	92
	1	225	54	75	6	245	55½	92
H. N.	7	202	50	73	6	215	57	69
	5	207	52	76	8	202	56	70
	2	217	49	79	7	209	58	70
	3	207	55	78	7	206	53	78
R. W.	4		57	60	6	227	56	75
	5		58	60	7	225	55	74
	3		58½	61	5	212	49	88
	4		55	60	4	215	56½	88
D. C.	3	197	38	74	5	185	30½	67
	8	185	38	79	9	195	40	72
	7	202	40	80	4	199	27½	68
	4	174	38	75	4	189	35	73
M. D.	6		55	80	6	232	55	85
	0		58½	83	7	235	55½	80
	4		56	83	6	241	55½	86
	8		55½	84	5	247	56	83
P. N.	7	214	48	73	6	224	49	73
	8	208	48	66	10	201	49	76
	6	213	48	78	7	210	47	78
	3	211	51	69	3	221	49½	81
H. P.	6	223			6	253	55½	62
	7	238			8	241	54½	56
	5	246			4	250	57½	55
	4	263			3	241	55	55

TABLE I (*continued*)

Name	First Records				Last Records			
	Rank	Tap-ping	Grip	Pulse	Rank	Tap-ping	Grip	Pulse
D. S.	8	216	65½	87	6	225	73½	70
	8	207	70	81	9	231	75	77
	9	216	67	80	7	227	75½	77
	9	221	66	81	9	238	74½	76
C. S.	8	225	71	80	8	220	68	76
	7	246	78½	80	7	227	72	76
	7	240	78½	85	5	244	77	77
	6	228	80	84	6	230	75	77
H. H.	3	174	48	80	5	209	48½	83
	3	176	49½	84	4	208	50	83
	6	185	51	83	3	206	46½	81
	7	201	50	79	4	201	46½	82
O. S.	2		53	69	6	208	45	82
	5		51	73	7	193	43	79
	6		55	76	4	184	48	79
	4		51	74	8	184	46	80
J. W.	6	231	59	84	4		60	88
	3	222	56	82	4		58	86
	8	210	62	80	8		58½	85
	8	187	62½	87	7		59	88
Average	5·88	207·3	53·4	73·8	6·09	216·4	55·4	74·5
	5·60	208·7	54·0	73·9	6·94	212·3	56·5	73·6
	5·00	212·8	54·9	76·6	4·91	213·3	55·9	75·8
	4·37	209·1	54·5	75·7	4·50	216·6	54·0	76·1

If now we examine the averages of first records at the end of the table we find that Beethoven with 5·88 and Tschaikowsky with 5·60 out of a possible ten points have an initial advantage in enjoyment value over the fox-trot with 5·00 and the one-step with 4·37. The two classical pieces are thus ranked about 22 per cent higher at the outset by this particular group of subjects. By the end of the twenty-fifth hearing this difference had risen to 38 per cent, as the Beethoven rating had risen to 6·09, and the Tschaikowsky rating to 6·94, while the jazz ranks had remained practically constant. The initial tapping record after hearing Beethoven was 207·3 and after Tschaikowsky was 208·7, an average of 208 taps per thirty seconds. The average of the two popular pieces was 211 taps, three more than for the classical music. For the fifty-one subjects who began the experiment there was an initial difference of six taps in favour of the popular music. At the end of twenty-five hearings this difference had almost entirely disappeared.

The records of the strength of grip, indicated in the third and seventh columns tell very much the same story as the tapping test. At first there is a difference of 1 kgm. or about 2 per cent in favour of the effect of jazz on this type of muscular performance. The difference was as much as 3·3 per cent for the original fifty-four subjects. But the column 7 records show that twenty-five repetitions had eliminated this initial difference, and had even left a slight advantage in favour of the classical selections. A test of steadiness given with a Bryan tracing board and an electric sounder resulted in initial scores of 7·6 and 7·0 for the original fifty-four subjects as they listened to the classical selections. The scores of these same subjects were better by 8 per cent when the jazz music was playing. As this test could be given only at the beginning of the experiment, no data appear under this head in the table, but it gave further evidence of a definite initial advantage in motor innervation resulting from the hearing of jazz music. Presumably the effect of constant repetition would have been to greatly reduce this difference.

The records in columns 4 and 8 show that the first hearing of a jazz selection gives the pulse 2·5 more beats per minute than does the first hearing of a classical selection. And this difference, curiously enough, seems not to disappear with the repetition of the selection.

The last comparison was that of the effects of the two

kinds of music on facial expression and bodily posture. Small groups of subjects were photographed while listening to each of the four selections and were told to give their attention to the music unmindful as far as possible of the fact that they were being photographed. The first two photographs show pictures of two groups as they listened for the first time to the two classical selections. The next two show the same persons listening for the first time to the two jazz records. Exact quantitative comparison is impossible here, but a close inspection of the photographs reveals some interesting contrasts of attitude. In listening to the unfamiliar classical music there is distinctly more tendency to lower the head, to avert the gaze, and to assume a slightly puzzled, uncomprehending expression. There is also considerably less tendency towards smiling lines about the mouth. A comparison of the last two sets of photographs presents quite a different contrast. Again we have two identical groups of subjects, but photographed in this case while listening for the twenty-fifth time. Note the greater erectness of posture, the greater directness of gaze, and other subtler evidences of interest are definitely in favour of the classical records. So far as the photographic evidence goes it tends to show that familiarization with classical music produces an attitude favourable to the best type of morale, whereas familiarization with jazz makes for a listless attitude. Briefly, the question raised by the camera in regard to music is whether it is better to go from a condition of puzzled strain to one of alert attention or from one of comprehending levity to one of bored listlessness. The question is a pointed one as regards phonograph records, for repetition is the inevitable rule with everything pertaining to the phonograph.

Conclusions

The data here presented tend to show that an unselected group of college undergraduates inclines to prefer the best classical music to the average jazz selection. And this preference increases rapidly as the two types of selection are repeated again and again. Indeed the experiment was seriously endangered at one time by repeated threats of a few of the subjects that they would break the jazz records if they were to be required to listen to them many more times. It is not, however, so evident that the twenty-five hearings made the group as a whole love jazz less, but rather that it made them love Beethoven and Tschaikowsky more.

Jazz records evidence their peculiar fitness for dancing by the greater motor innervation which they occasion, and by the more rapid pulse count that accompanies them. They also inspire a becoming levity of countenance most favourable to certain types of social occasion. But repetition is decidedly more favourable to the classical selection, whether we approach the comparison from the standpoint of enjoyment, of motor innervation or of facial expression.

Two educational conclusions seem to be implied by our results. The first is that since the strongly marked rhythm of street music has such an immediate stimulating value, it is important to select as our first music for the child of the musically immature pieces that have a strongly marked rhythm, as well as melodic, harmonic, or structural merit. It is the rhythm that will first get the child's spontaneous attention, and the other musical values will gradually unfold themselves to him as he hears the selection repeatedly. The second conclusion is that since good music apparently tends to develop interest when it is heard repeatedly with an unprejudiced mind, it is important not to inject any moral controversy into the matter of appreciating music. If a boy is faced with a piece of classical music that is slightly beyond his comprehension, and told that unless he enjoys it there is something wrong with him, he may easily set up defence mechanisms against all classical music. But though we may find that it does not pay to take a moralizing attitude in the teaching of good music, we should not lose sight of the ultimate fact suggested by our photographs, that the appreciation of good music does tend to make for improved morale. The great seriousness with which the Germans took their group music was the occasion of much amused comment during the early months of the war ; but one can hardly question now that music was used to better psychological effect by them than by either the French or the British. And the rôle of music in time of war has after all much in common with its rôle in time of peace. Seriousness of mind in crowds is a rare phenomenon without the aid of music, and it is becoming increasingly evident that serious crowd purposes are as insistently needed at present as they were even in August, 1914.

The superficial commercial argument from our data might perhaps be that it would be of more profit to the manufacturer of records to put his main emphasis on the type of selection for which the appeal will shortly decline, in the hope that new curiosity for other pieces may keep up the most continuous kind of demand. Against this stands the consideration that the purchaser who has grown fond of a classical selection will pay much more for the record that he so strongly desires ; and the further consideration that the man who has found durable pleasures in the field of phonograph music is likely to be more curious about exploring the whole field further. The influence of fashion in musical tastes is undoubtedly a great factor in altering temporarily the enjoyment values of certain kinds of pieces, but inasmuch as all fashions are temporary, we may fairly assume that the progress of enjoyment as described in a laboratory experiment is characteristic of the long-run effects on music from decade to decade. We may infer then that the manufacturer who expects to develop a steady, regular trade, in which he will supply the highest grade of workmanship is more justified in selecting classical music for the reason that these records will continue to make their appeal, and hence will constantly tempt the purchaser to explore new possibilities in the field.

CHAPTER XII

THE EFFECT ON A MUSICAL PROGRAMME OF FAMILIARITY
AND OF SEQUENCE OF SELECTIONS

JUNE E. DOWNEY AND GEORGE E. KNAPP

ONE of several definitions of music describes it as the art of expressing thought in tone. If we accept this statement as a premise, we may say that tone, which is sound regulated to definite pitch, can be made to express thought ; and the way in which tone is made to express thought is the basis for Musical Form.

In order that music may convey the thought which inspired the composer, it is necessary that the listener have some foundation for appreciation, whether in his training, experience, or native endowment ; and the way in which music may be considered by the listener is the basis for Musical Appreciation.

To an observer whose eye is trained, forms of architecture are recognizable and can be described intelligently. To a listener whose ear is trained, forms of music are recognizable, and can be described intelligently. To the untrained eye, forms of architecture may produce some emotional reactions which can be described only with incoherence. To the untrained ear, forms of music, likewise, may produce effects which cannot coherently be explained.

The experiment described in this chapter was conducted with a view to recording in numerical form the effects produced by repetition of a programme of musical compositions in varied order upon the individuals in a class of college students. The compositions were played on a phonograph, the records being chosen to represent the principal forms of music.

In the book " What We Hear in Music ", by Anne Shaw Faulkner-Oberndorfer, there are outlined four fundamental ideas which music can express. These are :

National Feeling : Patriotism, Occupations of the People, Folk-Dances.

Poetic Thought : Religion, Love, Happiness, Tranquillity, etc.

Programme Music : Imitation in Music, Grief, Humour, etc.

Formal Construction : March, Dance Forms, Sonata, etc,

Using this division as a basis for classification, compositions were selected, ten in all, which were grouped as follows :

National Feeling :

(a) Marche Slave—Tschaikowsky—Orchestra.

(b) Columbia, The Gem of the Ocean—D. T. Shore—Military Band.

Poetic Thought :

(a) Meditation from "Thais"—Massenet—Violin Solo.

(b) Kathleen Mavourneen—Crouch—Violin, 'Cello, and Piano.

Programme Music :

(a) Overture to " A Midsummer Night's Dream "—Mendelssohn—Concert Orchestra.

(b) Dream Pictures—Lumbye—Band.

(c) In a Clock Store—Orth—Concert Orchestra.

Formal Construction :

(a) Pomp and Circumstance—Elgar—Band.

(b) Invercargill March—Lithgow—Band.

Unclassified :

Cantonese Song—Chinese—Voice and Chinese Orchestra.

It will be noticed in the programme as listed above that the first number of each of the first four groups is the more subtle or involved example of the form it represents, while the second number is the most obvious example that could be found. In one group, that under programme music, three selections were listed, the third number being an exceptionally strong descriptive composition. In addition to the classified groups the record of the Chinese song was played in order to obtain some record of responses from dissonance and irregular time, in strong contrast to the melodious and orderly selections in the four groups.

The appeal to the listeners was made solely through rhythm, melody, and harmony, no vocal selections being used which could suggest moods other than those caused by absolute music. The Chinese record is partly vocal, but was not understandable by anyone in the class.

The musical programme outlined above was given in the Music Studio at weekly intervals (8 o'clock every Tuesday morning) for five weeks. The auditors were thirty-three students in psychology, all of some and a few of considerable training in psychological observation. Only three of the group had more than a passing acquaintance with music. The Seashore tests for musical talent showed the group to be, on the whole, of average or less than average musical ability.

The order of presentation for the different groups of selections was varied according to a definite procedure, except for the Cantonese Song, which was always put last and not included at all in the third programme. The first presentation conformed to the programme outlined above : the National Feeling group first. For the three following programmes each group was shifted up one place ; the first group going to fourth place. Within each group the *subtle* and *obvious* selections were alternated as part of the shift in order. The fifth order of arrangement was as follows : Thais, Midsummer Night's Dream, Marche Slave, Pomp and Circumstance, Kathleen Mavourneen, Dream Pictures, Invercargill March, Columbia, and In a Clock Shop.

For each programme the auditors were furnished with a record blank similar to the one reproduced below. A pause followed each musical number to permit recording the affective judgment and the imaginal response.

SAMPLE RECORD BLANK

Name—M.A. Date, 5th April, 1921 Mood Peevish Physical Condition Good

Selection	1	2	3	4	5	6	7	8	9	10
Familiar ? Where heard ? .		yes school					yes		yes	
4. Very, very pleasant .										
3. Very pleasant .	—	—	—				—		—	
2. Moderately pleasant					—					
1. Slightly pleasant					—	—		—		
0. Indifferent										
1. Slightly unpleasant .										—
2. Moderately unpleasant										
3. Very unpleasant										
4. Very, very unpleasant										
3. Very vivid			—				—		—	—
2. Moderately vivid										
1. Faint	—	—			—	—		—		
0. None										
Visual	—				—	—	—		—	—
Auditory	—				—		—		—	—
Motor			—				—		—	—
Miscellaneous								—		
Name of selection .		Columbia the Gem of the Ocean								

Preceding the first programme, the following instructions were given : " You are to hear a. number of musical selections. Mark your responses to each one by putting a dash in the proper squares. You are to make three reports : first, on the degree of pleasantness or unpleasantness of the selection you heard ; and second, and third, on the vividness and quality of imagery it aroused. Detailed introspections may be given on a separate sheet."

Included among other entrances on the record blank was a statement whether or not each selection was a familiar one and if so, whether its name was known.

Every suggestion that the same compositions were to be heard on successive Tuesdays was avoided so that it was possible to tell when the selection took on the *familiarity* character.

The following summary shows the extent to which each selection was recognized as *familiar* on the first day. The name was not necessarily known.

Columbia 33,

Invercargill March, 29 . . .	Recognized by all as familiar on second hearing.
Thais, 21	Not recognized by all as familiar until the fourth hearing.
Cantonese Song, 11 . .	Recognized by all as familiar on the second hearing.
Kathleen Mavourneen, 9 .	Not recognized by all as familiar until third hearing.
Pomp and Circumstance, 7 .	Not recognized by all as familiar until fourth hearing.
Marche Slave, 6 . . .	Not recognized by all as familiar until fourth hearing.
Dream Pictures, 3 . .	Not recognized by all as familiar until third hearing.
Midsummer Night's Dream, 2	Not recognized by all as familiar until fourth hearing.

As no names were given to the selections during the experiment, the title did not influence results greatly.

Table I gives in convenient form a numerical summary of affective judgments entered on the record blanks. For each selection, for each of the five days, an algebraic sum was obtained which represented the total affective response to that composition. Totals are also given for the five hearings of each selection ; and a total which represents the affective response for each day on all compositions taken together. The numbers in parentheses indicate the position on the programme of each selection for the different experimental sessions.

Inspection of this table reveals a number of interesting facts :

(1) The preferred selections were Kathleen Mavourneen, Invercargill March, and Thais. The preferred group that of Poetic Thought.

(2) The least preferred selections were Midsummer Night's Dream, Marche Slave, and Pomp and Circumstance. The least preferred group that of National Feeling.

(3) The Cantonese Song was felt to be definitely unpleasant. A few persons complained that an anticipation of hearing it operated to reduce their enjoyment of the programme as a whole.

(4) Except for the second programme there was continuous increase in the total pleasantness of the musical responses.

(5) In general, all of the selections participated in the increased pleasantness, but somewhat unequally.

The greatest increase in pleasantness is evident for the following compositions :

(a) Midsummer Night's Dream.
(b) Pomp and Circumstance.
(c) Dream Pictures.
(d) Kathleen Mavourneen.
(e) Thais.

Within each group, except Poetic Thought, the *subtle* composition gained more by repetition than did the obvious composition. The composition of highest æsthetic value gained most of all.

Only one number decreased in affective value, from the first to the fifth hearing, namely Columbia.

The general conclusion suggested by the table is that repetition within the limits of the present experiment operated definitely to increase the pleasantness of hearing these musical selections and that, relatively, the more *subtle* or æsthetic compositions gained the most by repetition. In a very long series of tests it would be possible to discover whether in time the compositions of the greatest artistic value would come to be strongly preferred even by non-musical persons to those less artistic, and whether obvious compositions would entirely cease to please.

TABLE I.—AFFECTIVE VALUE OF MUSICAL NUMBERS. 25 Persons

Programme.	I.	II.	III.	IV.	V.	Total.	Gain or loss (I–V).
National Feeling							
Marche Slave	41 (1)	25 (9)	28 (6)	43 (4)	42 (3)	179	+ 1
Columbia .	63 (2)	56 (8)	57 (7)	65 (3)	52 (8)	293	— 11
Totals .	104	81	85	108	94	472	
Poetic Thought							
Thais	62 (3)	61 (2)	67 (8)	61 (6)	78 (1)	329	+ 16
Kathleen Mavourneen .	68 (4)	77 (1)	82 (9)	84 (5)	87 (5)	398	+ 19
Totals .	130	138	149	145	165	727	
Programme Music							
Midsummer Night's Dream	19 (5)	17 (5)	50 (1)	53 (7)	63 (2)	202	+ 44
Dream Pictures .	46 (6)	50 (4)	62 (3)	60 (9)	67 (6)	285	+ 21
In a Clock Shop .	51 (7)	55 (3)	62 (2)	64 (8)	61 (9)	293	+ 10
Totals .	116	122	174	177 ·	191	780	
Formal Construction			*8 (4)				
Pomp and Circumstance	22 (8)	27 (7)	8 (4)	43 (2)	42 (4)	142	+ 24
Invercargill March	78 (9)	70 (6)	80 (5)	74 (1)	82 (7)	384	+ 4
Totals .	100	97	88	117	124	526	
Cantonese Song .	−68 (10)	−64 (10)		−62 (10)	−60 (10)	−254	+ 8
Total omitting Cantonese Song .	450	438	496	547	574		

* Instrument ran down.

The way in which repetition operates to increase the pleasantness of musical compositions will be considered in more detail later. At this point attention is called to the fact that Table I shows that while *familiarity* is a very considerable factor in determining the numerical totals, it is not the only factor.

Affective contrasts also influence the numerical ratings of the different musical selections.

For each of the first four programmes a different group of selections was placed first. Table I shows that this order of hearing had its effect. Undoubtedly, in the passing of judgments of pleasantness—unpleasantness, the standard of reference is a shifting one : probably the first selections constitute the standard by reference to which later ones are evaluated.

The most definitely preferred group in the present experiment was the Poetic Thought group. This group of compositions was placed first on the second programme and set the standard of evaluation for that day, with the result that there was a fall in the total affective value. It is probably more effective to have a pleasantness rated on an ascending scale rather than on a descending scale.

The same thing is shown from the other side by noticing the total values for the National Feeling, or least preferred group, when it stood first and last on the programme. In the second case contrast had its most deleterious effect, so far as the Marche Slave was concerned.

In the fifth programme where the *subtle* compositions were given first and then the *obvious* ones, it is likely that still greater increase in the affective total would have been found by placing Thais fourth instead of first and Kathleen Mavourneen ninth.

Table I also suggests that, other things being equal, a position midway of the programme is less advantageous than one at beginning or end of it.

In planning a programme for artistic effect or for training for musical appreciation the audience would need to be considered carefully. A highly popular number should not be given early in the programme. With an audience musically uncultured a light " encore " may serve to decrease the affective rating of less *obvious* sequent numbers. With a musically cultured audience an occasional light selection may enhance the value of more æsthetic selections. In training for musical appreciation a careful study should be made of affective contrasts. In the experiment under discussion, the effect of placing the Cantonese Song first should have been tried.

The auditors in the reported investigation were asked to keep records of the kind and vividness of their imaginal responses to the musical numbers as a crude indication of the effect of repetition upon the potency of the imagery aroused and of the influence of imagery-arousing music upon sequent numbers.

Table II summarizes the results in numerical form. Each record of the presence of an image was multiplied by 3, 2, 1, depending upon the degree of vividness entered on the chart and the totals obtained.

The chart records represent an unanalyzed mass of material. The consistency of the individual records indicate, however, the carefulness with which the report was made and the practice in observing images which the group as a whole had. It is not, however, likely that the hearers succeeded in any degree in distinguishing imaginal from actually sensational experience. In the case of reports of motor material there is, probably, a failure to distinguish very accurately incipient movements from motor images, but the grosser overt movements, such as tapping of the feet, movements of the hand and head, would be readily eliminated. The same assertion might be made for organic processes.

Table II gives the imaginal totals and the visual and motor value of each selection for each programme; the per cent. of motor and of visual process for each musical composition; and the rating of the selections for imaginal potency and for pleasantness.

To summarize :

(1) The most strongly imaginal selections were the Invercargill March, Columbia, and In a Clock Shop; the most strongly visual, In a Clock Shop, Invercargill March, and Columbia.

(2) The least imaginal numbers were Pomp and Circumstance, Dream Pictures and Marche Slave; the least visual, Pomp and Circumstance, Midsummer Night's Dream, and Marche Slave.

(3) There was, relatively, much motor material aroused by the Invercargill March, Pomp and Circumstance, and Columbia; little by Kathleen Mavourneen, Midsummer Night's Dream, or Thais. The strongly accented rhythms were more productive of a motor response, actual or imaged, which was frequently translated into visual terms.

(4) The unpleasantness of the Cantonese Song operated many times to inhibit a response. That frequently the selection was simply thrust out of consciousness is evident from the numerous cases in which no record is made for this selection apart from the fact of its great unpleasantness; there is a failure to enter even a negative response.

(5) The totals for imagery reveal a less constant effect due to familiarity than was evident on the affective side. There is, however, evidence of increasing visual material with some decrease in motor material. Possibly there is a growing tendency to translate motor reactions into the subtler optical-motor form.

TABLE II.—IMAGINAL POTENCY

Programme	I.			II.			III.			IV.			V.			Totals.	Motor %	Order Imaginal Potency.	Gain I–V.	Affective Order.
	V.¹	M.²	Total	V.¹	M.²	Total	V.¹	M.²	Total	V.¹	M.²	Total	V.¹	M.²	Total					
Imagery																				
National Feeling																				
Marche Slave	35	15	58	15	7	25	17	7	32	33	9	49	38	20	69	233	24	7·5	+11	8
Columbia	48	31	101	43	35	90	46	32	98	45	41	113	42	27	90	492	33	2	−11	4·5
Poetic Thought																				
Thais	27	13	58	32	5	47	35	20	62	33	7	45	40	9	56	288	20	6	−2	3
Kathleen Mavourneen	31	5	44	21	2	29	41	5	66	45	8	58	55	14	89	286	12	5	+45	1
Programme Music																				
Midsummer Night's Dream	18	10	43	22	9	36	22	4	31	31	5	45	35	11	61	216	18	9	+18	7
Dream Pictures	29	26	69	34	23	67	30	22	67	36	10	67	40	19	71	341	28	4	+2	6
In a Clock Shop	41	25	88	57	33	108	59	26	108	57	17	97	40	15	68	469	24	3	−20	4·5
Formal Construction																				
Pomp and Circumstance	12	10	29	15	15	35	22	7	33	20	14	37	38	15	57	191	32	10	+28	9
Invercargill March	40	40	96	57	52	120	47	39	111	42	28	89	53	50	126	542	39	1	+30	2
Total, omitting Cantonese Song	281	75	586	296	181	557	319	162	608	342	139	600	381	180	687					

¹ Visual.   ² Motor.

The different selection gave, however, different results so far as imaginal material was concerned. There is some indication of an increase in imaginal responses for the more *subtle* selection and of decrease for the more *obvious* ones. Comparing the records for Programmes I and V, it appears that Kathleen Mavourneen, Invercargill March, Pomp and Circumstance, Midsummer Night's Dream, and Marche Slave show considerable gain in imaginal potency; there is practically no change for Thais, Dream Pictures, and the Cantonese Song; some decrease for In a Clock Shop and Columbia.

(6) The ratings for affective value and for imaginal potency indicate no very close relationship.

It was thought in planning the experiment that the imaginal totals might be extensively affected by the selections placed at the beginning of the programme. For one of the writers of the paper this is so definitely the case that a musical composition strongly visual in its suggestions may set the response to a whole programme. Since programme music is for her most apt to be visual in content, there was anticipated increased imagery, particularly visual imagery, on the day when the programme-music was placed first, namely, the third day. The imaginal total for this day is high, but not as high as on the fifth day and practically the same as on the fourth day. The selection placed first, Midsummer Night's Dream, was, however, not imaginally potent for the class as a whole. The group most potent in arousing motor processes when placed first, served possibly to actually decrease motor response to sequent selections.

A new factor operated in the later programmes, namely memory of images previously experienced. With growing familiarity with a composition such imaginal effects are for certain persons cumulative; others record a feeling of latent imagery. For another and less flexible type of person there is a stereotyping of imagery, quite similar to the stereotyping of backgrounds found in literary responses.

The relation of familiarity, affective contrasts, and imaginal responses to musical enjoyment is a very complex one. The introspective notes of the class reveal some interesting tendencies. But instead of tabulating them, the notes of one expert listener, not included in the tabular summary, are produced in part.

For this person there is a very great interest in novel effects. A rapid waning in pleasantness accompanies repetition of a composition unless the music is very rich and complex.

Excerpts from the reports for the five days are given below :—

Programme I. Greatly interested in test : Good physical condition. Selections all familiar.

Most complete absorption in Thais. Turned away from group ; complete detachment. No imaginal response.

Greatest amount of imagery for Programme-Music Group. Dream Pictures produced more imaginative material than In a Clock Shop. The images aroused by latter were memory images, often with a definite temporal reference.

Mood became definitely objective and matter-of-fact during the playing of the Invercargill March ; Park-Mood ; noticed the movements and attitudes of the class.

Cantonese Song was slightly pleasant because of the curiosity it aroused. Some of the intervals are interesting.

Programme II. Objective, alert, scientific attitude : excellent physical condition.

Almost no tendency to become absorbed in music : found programme pleasant because of general pleasantness of mood. Attention centred on tone, melody, rhythm, and structure : very little emotional or imaginal appeal.

In a Clock Shop. Moderately pleasant, due to detached pleasantness of tones and to restful sounds, not to composition of selection. Did not get the wealth of visual material noticed the week before although I *remembered* it. Very faint visual glimpses of man winding clock and faint glimpse of big clock face. Many associative ideas and words. Stevenson's story (what's the name ?) and memory (with atmosphere toning) of evening in a Chicago Art-Gallery with many chiming clocks in the neighbourhood, and the words " Cuckoo ! " and " Whistling ! " Verbal Description of what each representation was of. Affective, not æsthetic pleasantness.

Dream Pictures, moderately pleasant. No imaginal response, although I recall memory of pictures previously imaged ; these images just below the threshold of attention and would emerge if I wanted them. Concentrate instead on the *tempo*, which seems faster than I remembered it and on the melody which in previous hearing of selection was only an accompaniment to the pictures. This is my third hearing of the composition, which is definitely waning in value. Cloyingly sweet.

Columbia. Slightly pleasant at first ; then moderately unpleasant because of fourfold repetition of melody. At first just an accompaniment to drifting thought. Then became insistent and unpleasant.

Marche Slave. Moderately pleasant ; interesting ; a relief from the monotony of preceding record. But record itself disappointing.

Cantonese Song. Moderately pleasant. I like the rhythm and the organic effect of certain tones and glides.

Programme III. Clear bright mood, but eyes fatigued from lack of sleep, which probably increased the amount of visual imagery. The initial programme-music also gave a *visual* set to consciousness.

Dream Pictures. Visual-motor images of dancing fairies ; visualization is largely of filmy floating draperies and sinuous figures advancing and retreating. Flower-bells seen, large white bells, luminous in the moonlight and swaying in the breeze. At final movement fairies arise from the flower-bells and dance again.

Some lovely waltz and march effects and at one place a delightfully staccato reversal of movement; and advance and retreat of fairies with military precision.

Columbia. The repetition of the theme is intolerable. Four times! I can't stand it! Attention wanders.

Programme IV. Mood composed, cheerful. Physical condition good.

Marche Slave. Fits organic tempo but fails to hold attention.

Invercargill March. Just an accompaniment of my thoughts.

Columbia. Just an accompaniment to thought of WHY DO I DISLIKE REPETITION OF A THEME SO EXTREMELY?

Marche Slave. Contrast to Columbia. Very pleasing; so much more interesting; but intervals did not harmonize with organic *set*.

Kathleen Mavourneen. Complete kinæsthetic relaxation; tones are lovely; change in mood and set.

Thais. More exciting than preceding selection; quickened breathing and pulse.

Midsummer Night's Dream. Lovely pictures; dancing fairies and dancing motes in sunlight. Forest pierced with shaft of light; darkness seen and felt.

Dream Pictures. Too familiar and all-explored; no dance mood as before.

Cantonese Song.—Interesting, but made head ache.

Programme V. Bad physical condition. Fagged; strung-up, organic tension, very conscious of heart-beat. Believe I am in a definite *key*.

Thais. Off organic *key*. Irritated me.

Midsummer Night's Dream. Time and *key* better suited to organic condition.

Marche Slave. Exactly my *key* this morning. Did not feel disappointed in record as before.

Pomp and Circumstance. First and last part made heart-beat too apparent to be pleasing; middle part induced relaxation.

Kathleen Mavourneen. Relieved tension somewhat.

Dream Pictures. Unpleasantly conscious of heart-beat ; agreeable associations.

Invercargill March. Accentuated heart-beat greatly ; too bright, measured and monotonous.

Columbia. Have been dreading this in anticipation. Allowed attention to be distracted by thoughts on the *Therapeutic Value of Music.* Music served fairly well as an accompaniment to this prosaic theme.

Cantonese Song. Very exciting and *frightfully* interesting. " Hurt Heart."

As a whole the music improved physical condition ; it is, however, evident that if music is to be used for therapeutic purposes, some very exacting studies will be necessary.

The relation of familiarity and novelty to the æsthetic response has been approached from a number of different angles.

With respect to the art product itself it has been shown that power to maintain its pleasing quality is one indication of real æsthetic value. But why should the æsthetic gain on the merely pleasing from greater familiarity with it ? This brings us to the question of the individual, who responds to the art product.

Familiarity is in itself a pleasant feeling ; it involves the *recognitive thrill* which is in part a feeling of safety, of being *at home.* So strong a factor in toning a situation may mere familiarity be that even a personal enemy seen in a strange environment may be welcomed, as beautifully exemplified in the story of the southern feudist who left his native haunts to seek his enemy, intending to " shoot on sight ", but who, overcome with delight on seeing a familiar face in the wilderness of a great city, indulged in an embrace instead of a murder ! With too great acquaintance, however, familiarity lapses into triteness and pleasingness washes out. The only protection against such waning in value is a very rich content in the object.

Novelty is a second factor which forces attention and brings in train the joy of adventure. In order that the *familiar* may not pass over into the *trite*, its content must be so rich, so complex, as to insure continued discovery of new beauties, or subtleties not to be grasped from one presentation. But a variational factor in individuals operates here to further complicate the situation. With certain persons, familiarity is so potent a factor that everything departing from the accustomed is felt to be grotesque, disagreeable. Because strange it is unpleasant, an unpleasantness which may obliterate the real elements of beauty. For such individuals all highly original productions of art or of nature will be disagreeable, just because new. No new art-feature will be appreciated until its unaccustomedness has worn away. For other persons the new or strange or bizarre has an obsessive value which gives them a thrill not to be obtained from the old and familiar. Such persons make haste to welcome novel movements in art, hail each new school of poetry or painting as supreme.

The varying value for different individuals of novelty and familiarity has long been recognized by writers on æsthetics, particularly in connexion with their discussions of the classic and romantic temperament. But from the psychological side little effort has been made to identify the factors that operate to place an individual in one group or the other. A profitable suggestion appears in an investigation by Myers and Valentine [1] :

[1] " A Study of the Individual Differences in Attitude towards Tones," *Brit. Journal of Psychology*, vol. vii.

" The influence of familiarity on appreciation is most marked in subjects who make frequent use of the associative aspect, while that of strangeness is most marked in those who make frequent use of the conative sub-aspect and the objective aspect. Familiarity has a positive effect when the associative is combined with the conative sub-aspect, and a negative effect when the associative is combined with the physiological sub-aspect."

The aspects referred to in the quoted paragraph are those recognized by Bullough and the writers of the article as characterizing the responses of individuals to sensory content. Four main aspects of perceptual responses are recognized (a) the intra-subjective aspect ; (b) the objective aspect ; (c) the character aspect and (d) the associative aspect. Under the intra-subjective aspect there are a number of sub-aspects, two of which are the physiological and the conative. The character aspect is the most intimately aesthetic. It is " not dependent on the intra-subjective or associative aspects, in nature and origin it is *sui generis* ". [1]

The character aspect of sensory material is stressed somewhat rarely. The introspective notes of the listeners of the present experiment indicate a very great emphasis of the associative aspect except by the one expert listener. Under such circumstances we may expect familiarity to operate in increasing pleasantness, as in fact it did.

An analysis of the introspective reports revealed the influence of the associative factors.

(1) Memorial images were frequently experienced ; glimpses of surroundings in which the composition had been heard previously ; or visualization of the instrument, the musician or the band that had played it. Memory

[1] See Chapter II.

of the whole situation in which it was heard operated to give the selection the connotation of a parade, a rally, a patriotic meeting, a social gathering and the like.

Sometimes the associations evoked by the music produced a common effect upon a number of auditors. Thus, in the Clock Shop record, there are many reports that an early morning scene is described, though there may be no memory of the time indicated by the striking of the clocks. Several insist that it should be six o'clock in the morning, although they think it two or four by the clocks !

(2) Stereotyping of images gave an increasingly reminiscent flavour for some persons.

(3) When the title was known this operated to call up associations in addition to those due to the stimulus of the music. The effect of the title in suggesting associations was amusingly shown in one case where the listener made a mistake in identifying a selection. The reverse side of the record, In a Clock Shop, is devoted to A Hunting Scene. The person had confused the two selections and reported rich imagery illustrative of hunting instead of the imagery so appropriately evoked by the Clock Shop record ! Those who knew the Cantonese Song by name reported at times Oriental Settings, the pleasantness of which overcame, in part, the tonal dissonances.

(4) Strongly accented time furnished a framework for motor classification of musical compositions, a possibility which enhances the pleasantness of strongly motor compositions.

(5) Anticipation of melodic phrases gave a feeling of mastery which increased the pleasure in hearing a composition.

The present investigation contributes somewhat to

R

an understanding of the course of development to be anticipated from repeated hearing of musical selections. The experiment should be carried out on musically cultured persons to discover how far a similar condition holds for them. Familiarity certainly increased the affective value of the more *subtle* musical compositions and might be counted upon as a factor in training in musical appreciation.

Further experiment in the making of programmes is necessary in order to determine in detail to what extent one may employ affective contrast in enhancing the pleasurableness of a particular composition or a whole programme.

SECTION VI

EFFECTS OF MUSIC BESIDES AUDITORY AND ORGANIC

Introductory Note.—Psychologists are still in disagreement concerning the senses that function most characteristically in the æsthetic experience. At one extreme are those who maintain that it is only the so-called higher senses, vision, and hearing, that are the true æsthetic senses, while at the other end of the scale are those who find the seat of the experience of beauty in the so-called lower senses, pain, temperature, equilibrium, kanæsthetic, and organic. Between these two extremes is the camp of those who steer a middle course and attribute to all senses a function in the appreciation of art.

The studies presented in this section are of much interest and value in that they indicate the part played in the musical experience of other senses than that of hearing. Both studies are very suggestive of further problems for research and investigation.—EDITOR.

CHAPTER XIII

NON-AUDITORY EFFECTS OF MUSIC

OTTO ORTMANN

IN discussing the non-auditory responses, the general psycho-physiological principles underlying the three stages [1]—sensorial, perceptual, and imaginal—need not be repeated. The analysis of these principles for audition, holds, in substance, for any other sensory field. Accordingly, whereas the auditory response is limited to one field, the non-auditory divides into the various non-auditory sense departments : visual, kinæsthetic, olfactory, and gustatory.

Of these, vision is, for our purposes, the most important. In its basic stage, the sensorial, two elements function : brightness and colour. The gold of the harp, the brilliant hue of the brass instruments, the soft grey light of the auditorium, the delicate pink of Mrs. Smith's new evening gown, are colour sensations that very few concert-goers do not receive. The list could readily be extended. Are these sensations lost ? Unfortunately, not at all ! They lead into visual perceptive responses just as auditory sensations lead into auditory perceptive responses. And with this development their importance in musical appreciation increases. The movements of the orchestral conductor, the facial expressions of the singer, the bowing of the violinist, and the key-attack of the pianist, are all visual stimulations. And the extent to which such factors determine our musical enjoyment, cannot be better illustrated than by facts such as the following :

[1] See Chapter III.

Of six musical persons, four of them professional musicians, four had decided not to attend the concerts of the Symphony Orchestra because the movements of the conductor destroyed their pleasure in the music. All admitted a reasonable artistic worth of the musical rendition. Yet in spite of the latter, the affective tone of the visual stimulus was sufficiently strong to counteract completely that of the auditory stimulus. Remarks such as " doesn't she look sweet ! " " his face is a study ", and the like, are known to every concert-goer and need no further explanation. I cannot refrain from appending an instance where visual reaction has had a deplorable effect. A blind violinist of merit quotes from a letter to his father from musical managers in England : " Don't bring your son to England ; the English public does not wish to see a blind man on the stage." The violinist had met a similar attitude in this country.

In order to ascertain in a general way the ratio of auditory response to non-auditory in the normal concert audience, a count was taken as follows : Unselected members of the audiences were observed sufficiently long for their attitude to be fairly well ascertained : whether they were listening entirely or were using their eyes during the rendition of the music. Doubtful cases were excluded. Only those cases were counted as pure auditory in which all use of the eyes was absent. Since the type of response of any individual changes, as we have seen, this method of procedure introduces an error. However, since counts were taken at three different concerts, and were not restricted to any one part of the audience, this error is a compensating, and not a cumulative one. The results obtained, allowing again for any doubtful cases, still showed less than 4 per cent of pure auditory response and approximately 90 per cent of visual response. Of course, this visual response does not necessarily exclude auditory response, but it does mean that *visual* impressions were received, and hence reacted to.

Another proof of the extent of visual responses is found in the sale of tickets for piano recitals. The pianist invariably sits so that many persons on the right side of the hall (facing the stage) cannot see the keyboard nor the artist's hands. If seeing the keyboard and the hands plays a part in our musical enjoyment, we should expect more seats on the left side of the hall to be sold than on the right side ; or, if all are sold, that those on the left side are sold first. Inquiry brought to light the fact that this is true, without exception. In fact, the visual response has become so distinctly habitual that this left-side preference was found to apply also to three operatic performances, in which, of course, no visual advantage was derived. The request printed on the programmes of the symphony concerts : " Ladies are kindly requested to remove their hats " is not printed for acoustical reasons : nor is the turning on of the footlights, when the singer appears on the stage, intended to improve the voice.

And finally, the entire printed programme is a visual stimulant, from the simple *allegro giojoso* or *adagio patetico* or even from the unmodified *presto* or *lento* to the pages of notes minutely describing a modern tone-poem. An intelligent deaf person, versed in the Italian terminology, and watching the gestures of certain orchestral conductors, has no difficulty in distinguishing the slow music from the fast, the gentle from the vigorous, the graceful from the majestic, though not a sound be heard. An unmusical adult, who was a regular attendant at symphony concerts, was asked why she applauded enthusiastically an involved Strauss Tone-poem and not a Beethoven Symphony. " I'm not musical enough to appreciate Beethoven," she replied. " But the Tone-poem, after I have read the programme, gives me something to think about. I can picture and enjoy all the happenings, and do not need to follow the music so closely." This is a case of appreciation not of the music, but almost in spite of the music. And what is more is that, in a modified form, this response is typical of not a small portion of our symphony audiences.

Instances of non-auditory responses to the presentation of music are not restricted to vision. The mouldy stage smell, the burning incense in the oriental scene, the delicate (?) aroma of our perfumed neighbour, are not without effect upon our response to the music of the opera. Scriabin desires his Prometheus to be performed to the accompaniment of changing lights, and his Mystery, to the accompaniment not only of colours but also of odours, both of which, he believes, enhance the response.

Nor does such non-auditory response stop at the perceptual stage. It is often elaborated into an imaginal form which leads to complexes so remote from the actual music as to seem ludicrous. So long as these responses are analyzed by the individual, and properly classified as non-auditory responses, they fall beyond the scope of the present analysis. But often they are not thus analyzed, and are attributed, albeit in a vague sort of way, to the music itself. They then give rise to one form of reciprocal types, described later.

If now, we extend non-musical responses to include the spoken or sung *word*, as opposed to the purely tonal aspect, we broaden the field of non-tonal response considerably.   Many songs owe their effect not to the music, but to the words.   This is particularly true of many hymns of to-day.   All vocal music, opera, in fact any tonal utterance described by a single word, is to that extent not purely tonal.   The latter aspect of the art of music as practised to-day, is therefore reduced to a rather inconsiderable minimum.   There is, unfortunately, no purely tonal art.   A concert of so-called *absolute music*, strictly speaking, would have to be given in a lightless hall, without printed or announced programme. Such an experiment, carefully made, and compared with the usual form of concert presentation, would furnish unmistakable evidence of the widespread existence of non-auditory effects of music.   *A psychology of musical enjoyment will be adequate only when we cease to attribute to tonal sources the effects which take their rise in non-tonal fields.*

Thus far we have kept distinct the two main forms of response, the auditory and the non-auditory.   But, since we are dealing with the responses of a highly integrated organism, we find no clear definition of types actually existing.   Instead, auditory stimuli cause a response which may lead over, through associations, into non-auditory fields ; and non-auditory stimuli may cause a response which leads over into the auditory field.   The former constitutes the compound response-type ; the latter, the reciprocal response-type.

COMPOUND TYPES

Two truths force themselves upon the investigator of response-types early in the investigation.   The first is, that no psycho-physiological type is at any time abruptly and decisively separated from other types ; and the second is, that within each individual the type changes.

Consequently, not only does the sensorial effect lead gradually into the perceptual, and this, in turn, to the imaginal, but elements of the one are practically always present in the other. It is the central manifestation that determines the designation of type. Thus we may have a sensorial-perceptual auditory response, or a perceptual-imaginal auditory response, or any other combination of two or more of the processes involved. This interrelation is not limited to audition, but also connects the auditory with the non-auditory responses, producing the compound types.

Association between auditory and non-auditory sensation, produces, for instance, the sensorial-sensorial type. Synæsthesis, in its most elementary form, is an instance of this type of response. When a tone, or an unanalyzed chord, but not a tonality, suggests a mere colour, such as blue, red ; or a taste such as sour, sweet ; or a smell such as aromatic, alliaceous, the association is between two originally relatively fundamental sensations. Such associations are not infrequently met with. Thus to one person D. is dark brown, violet ; b— dark blue ; a—light blue ; a_1—ochre-yellow ; g_2—light yellow ; c_4—whitish yellow with a touch of rose ; other persons, in a more general way, find high pitches white, middle pitches grey, and low pitches black. In some cases, passing from low to high, the order of colour associations is : black, dark brown, brown-red, red, orange, yellow, white. In the subjects tested, colour synæsthesia was found in 28 per cent. Another subject, when the tones were given on the piano found E_1 to F_1, sweet ; g to c^4, banana ; c^4 to c^5, insipid.

This type of response extends further and results in perceptual re-innervation in non-auditory fields. Thus a person responding to the tone of a D tin whistle found it :

" like Christmas candy," and to the piano tones A_2 to E_1 " like toast, soaked in water ". In vision, when blue becomes " the blue of an October sky ", or when in smell, the sound suggests a " salt water river with river traffic ", we have not only a perceptual image (image of memory) but, probably, also a productive imaginal effect. These compound types may be called, for purposes of analysis, the sensorial-perceptual, and the sensorial-imaginal. An example of the latter is furnished by introspections such as the following : " I must have been dreaming. I was startled by a jolt, as if the train had started. I was sitting in a railroad coach, mapping out my next sales." The subject in this case was a salesman ; the jolt he received was probably a fortissimo chord, used in a relatively quiet environment. This chord constituted the sole auditory stimulus, and it was carried over immediately into a non-auditory field, moreover, into a field richest in association for this subject.   Again

the following chord :   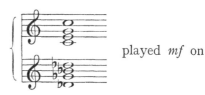   played *mf* on

the piano and allowed to diminish freely, produced the following responses in four pupils :—(1) " Just a sound. It does not mean anything. Not pretty, not ugly." (2) " Ugh ! I hate it ! Sounds all wrong ! "   (3) " Not specially nice. Could perhaps be used better with other chords."   (4) " I love it ! It reminds me of the 31st of December, when all the whistles are blowing at midnight." This last is an example of the sensorial-imaginal response.

A second class of compound response is that originating in the perceptual response of audition, and leading (through imagery) to the sensorial, perceptual, and imaginal responses in the non-auditqry field, and termed accordingly: the perceptual-sensorial; perceptual-perceptual; perceptual-imaginal. To the first of these complex responses belong those cases of synæsthesia in which tones of particular instruments or of particular tonalities awaken colour, taste, smell, or kinæsthetic sensations. One person (2) finds the tone of the 'cello, indigo blue; the human voice, green; the trumpet, red; the flute, scarlet; the violin and the viola, ultramarine; the clarinet, yellow; the oboe, rose-red; the french horn, purple; and the bassoon, violet. Other persons are affected differently. Of course, it is quite possible, in fact probable, that some of these associations are originally derived from non-auditory stimuli, in which case we have examples of reciprocal responses. But whatever the original association, whether auditorially initiated or not, it forms a compound type, one form of which is the reciprocal of the other; for every type which we are here considering has its reciprocal type in each other sensory field.

The type of response shown by the phenomenon of so-called characteristics of keys is an example of compound response. The particular type of this compound response depends upon the explanation which we adopt. The synæsthesic theory, according to which tonality suggests colours, tastes, or smells directly, makes it a perceptual or imaginal-sensorial response. The physiological theory, which explains the characteristics on the basis of physiological resonance of partials present in the clangs, makes it a sensorial-sensorial, or a sensorial-perceptual response. The vocal theory makes it a sensorial-sensorial response; the notation theory, a reciprocal response originating in the visual field; and, finally, the historical theory, which explains key-characteristics through the use of certain keys in well-known compositions, may make it a non-auditory response entirely. The exact compound-type can be determined only when the particular association-complex is known. If tonality or key is auditorally perceived, then the response begins with the auditory-perceptual type. If, on the other hand, the key is given in the programme, and the person responds on the basis of the historical theory, the reaction is entirely non-auditory. Thus, if a composition announced in E major awakens associations with fire through the non-auditory recall of Wagner's " Feuerzauber ", but not an image of the music, we have an example of a non-auditory response. Or if the key of C minor is known, but not through the ear, and suggests fate through the association with the Fifth Symphony of Beethoven, known to be in C minor, this, too, is a non-auditory response entirely.

As to the degree to which transfer from audition to non-audition takes place, it is difficult to make an estimate. In the imagery test, already referred to, which was given to several hundred persons, who were asked to give as many appropriate titles as possible to five short, characteristic compositions played on the piano, the approximate percentages of titles for each of the five, which showed auditory imagery unmistakably were 45%, 58%, 31%, 75%, and 45%. These figures are approximate only. In a group of six persons in which doubt as to the character of their imagery was removed by subsequent questioning, the percentages of auditory imagery for the same composition were: 18%, 63%, 9%, 78%, 58%. The percentile distribution given, coupled with the fact that the quantity of imagery of any kind varied from one piece to another, shows that neither the quantity nor the kind (auditory or non-auditory) of the imaginal response is fixed. Both are determined by the particular stimulus, and vary with the individual. Two specific cases may serve as illustrations. The first illustrates a change from 100% visual imagery to a 100% auditory imagery in the same subject. " The Little Nymphs," " The Beautiful Fairies," " Playday," " Dance of the Leaves," and for another composition " The Great Battle," " The Thunderstorm," " The Roaring of the Waves." The second case illustrates variation with the stimulus in richness of imagery. For the first composition : " Snowflakes," " Raindrops," " A Meadow Brook," " Woodland Sprites," and for the other composition : " Cradle Song." Or, from the replies of another person : " The Indian's Arrow," " The Flying Bird," " The Wizard," " The Toy Train," and for the other composition : " The Storm."

A third type of compound response is that originating in the imaginal-auditory response, and leading, through association, into one or more of the stages of the non-auditory field. Thus anticipation, or imaged variation of auditory stimuli by the listener, may suggest activities in non-audition. This type of response is not widespread, chiefly because its auditory basis itself represents a specialized main type of response. Physiologically it has a basis similar to the compound perceptual effects already described, with the difference that in the former the auditory stimulus is an image (subjective in origin) and in the latter it is a perception (objective in origin). The familiar observation of having a " tune running through my head ", if it leads to imagery in non-auditory fields is an example of the imaginal-imaginal effect. Non-auditory associations aroused by an original composition before this is *objectively* heard, are further instances ; and often suggest the title of a new work to the composer.

The compound responses leading to kinæsthesia should be emphasized on account of the important rôle that they play in musical effects. The nature of music demands reproduction for its appreciation. Reproduction involves technique, and technique means kinæsthesia. Kinæsthetic associations, therefore, are the dominating type for all instrumental performers. The particular type of kinæsthetic association depends upon the instrument used ; the singer will have vocal association, the pianist will have finger associations, and the horn player, lip associations. " I cannot see a phrase without feeling it in my fingers," is a familiar remark of good sight-readers. It is possible that such an association may not even touch the auditory field, although in most cases, the auditory image exists along with the visual and kinæsthetic images.

These are special types of kinæsthetic responses. When the latter are general, they give rise to what has been called the motor type of response. The auditory sources for this type are found not only in rhythm but in the outline described by melodic motion, and the strain and relaxation involved in dissonance and consonance, as well as in *crescendo* and *diminuendo*. And, since movement is, perhaps, the most effective of all musical elements, kinæsthetic sensations are a very important type of non-auditory response. They, like the visual, are far more usual than is generally admitted, and form the true basis of many responses that are daily traced to auditory sources.

RECIPROCAL TYPES

Finally, a few words should be said about what may be termed reciprocal types. If our analysis had been concerned primarily with some other sense department than audition, all the compound-types which have been described would become reciprocal types for that other sense department. In the compound types thus far described the original stimulus, in each case, is auditory. In the reciprocal types the original stimulus is non-auditory and leads over into audition in the same manner in which the auditory stimulus leads over into non-auditory fields. Accordingly, auditory imagery may be brought into play which is entirely at variance with the auditory stimulus actually present. To this class belong those cases, for example, in which a pathological condition of the listener results in a transfer of characteristics of bodily condition to the music. " The music was uninteresting, but then I was tired, and I'm not sure how much this influenced the music." Or from the reaction of a physically sub-normal child to a composition of rather bright character : " It seems to be telling a story of woe." Another person, listening to a peaceful Adagio, remarked that certain parts had had a " restless, scary, foreboding of evil " character. Subsequent questioning showed this character to have resulted from a fluttering heart, from which the subject was suffering. This connexion, however, was not suspected by the subject.

Other associations are those transferring visual or kinæsthetic form and movement to the auditory field. A certain motion suggests a certain melody ; a certain form suggests a certain composition. This type of response is the procedure followed when a landscape, a poem, or a dance inspires a musical composition. Examples of this type of response are well-known and not infrequent.

The presence of auditory imagery, therefore, is not

proof of a purely, or essentially, auditory response. Nor need we explain this imagery on auditory grounds. Thus, the entire mood of the music may be changed through non-auditory stimuli. At a song recital in which the singer stressed the histrionic aspect at the expense of all else, songs, the music of which was undoubtedly serious, assumed the character of gaiety and ludicrousness for many of the auditors. This resulted from a visual stimulation—the gestures and facial expression of the artist. The case of the orchestral conductor already cited, is a further illustration of the influence of a non-auditory stimulus upon auditory perception, and through that, upon musical enjoyment.

And this response type furnishes also the explanation of the all-too-frequent differences of opinion as to the real musical worth of a composition or a performance. A very small part of the audience goes to a concert in a musically unbiased attitude. And the greater the musical training, the greater the bias, usually. Like or dislike of a particular style of composition, national differences, petty jealousies, like or dislike of the social, ethical, or moral status of a musician all carry over, with telling effect, into the appreciation of that musician's purely musical attainments, and illustrate the reciprocal type of response. To this type belong also by far the greatest number of responses of our music critics, most of which cannot be explained on auditory ground.

The reciprocal types are compound-types. They differ from the other compound-types in their non-auditory origin ; and they differ from the non-auditory main response, which remains non-auditory, in their transfer of this origin to the auditory field.

CHAPTER XIV

A STUDY IN THE USE OF SIMILES FOR DESCRIBING MUSIC
AND ITS EFFECTS

ESTHER L. GATEWOOD

REPORTS of concerts and music reviews of various kinds
abound in descriptive terms which have little or no
relation to music itself. Many of them are terms
descriptive of sensations other than those of audition.
To call them figures of speech is not an explanation of
their use. Musicians and artists are particularly fond
of elaborate descriptions in such terms, while those who
are more prosaic minded often consider them merely
idealistic interpretations peculiar to temperamental
musicians. Does the use of such terms as bright, lyrical,
colourful, gay, graceful, mean anything, and if so, is
there a definite meaning attached to each term, so
definite that one can interpret objectively these terms
when used by various writers ?

The purpose of this study is to investigate the adequacy
of certain figurative expressions and the reliability and
consistency of their use. How universal is the tendency
to convert the enjoyment of music, either consciously
or unconsciously, into terms of other personal experiences?
Can such descriptive terms be classified into types or
groups ? Have they some organic characteristic or
relation ? Are they used consistently on different
occasions ?

An Edison laboratory model instrument was used to
reproduce the programme of musical selections. Eight

selections, representing types of music differing in rhythm, volume, instrumentation, tempo, were played. No vocal numbers were included. The selections were as follows :

> Volunteers' March (Sousa).
> Meditation—Thais (Massanet).
> On Wings of Song (Mendelssohn).
> Somewhere in Naples.
> Part I, Nut Cracker (Grieg).
> Norwegian Echo Song (Thrane).
> Humoresque (Dvorak).
> Ride of the Valkyries (Wagner).

Twelve young women, students of Columbia University, most of them advanced or graduate students, volunteered to listen in the experiment. The hour chosen was that immediately following dinner in the evening, a time which was usually devoted to recreation, often to music, in the dormitory. The young women were comfortably seated in the room, provided with data sheets (like the accompanying illustration), and instructed to listen until each musical number was finished, and at the close to record their descriptions without consultation or comparison of opinions.

The descriptive terms written on the data sheets are arranged in groups, the listeners being instructed to score one from each group, whichever one best fitted the music just heard. This method gives an objective means of comparison of the descriptions of several people. There were eight musical numbers on the first programme. These same selections were repeated, with the exception of one, the Overture Miniature, from the Nut Cracker Suite, after an interval of five days. The scorings from one hearing of the Overture Miniature are given in the last column of Table I. If a person felt that none of the terms of a given group fitted or described the selection just heard, she was to leave the whole space blank.

TABLE I.—TABLE SHOWING SELECTIONS ON WHICH THERE IS AGREEMENT IN TOTAL SCORING FOR TWO HEARINGS.

		80486 Volunteers' March	80243 Meditation—Thais	82236 On Wings of Song	50856 Somewhere in Naples	82230 Norwegian Echo Song	82228 Humoresque	80638 Ride of the Valkyries	80594 Nut Cracker—Part I
Size	large	30			30	30		30	
	small		20	0			0	20	30
Grey	black							30	
	white		20	0	0	20	30		20
Linear	straight lines	30			20			0	
	curved lines		30	30			30		30
Light	dark							30	
	light	20	0		30	0	30		20
Distance	far		0					0	
	near	20				30	20		0
Weight	light		20	0			30		30
	heavy							30	
Colour	red	0						30	
	orange								
	yellow								
	green								
	blue				0		0		
	violet			0					
Temperature	warm	30		30	30		30		30
	cold					0		30	
Taste	sour								
	sweet		30	30				20	
	salt	0				20			
	bitter								
Movement	movement	30			30		0	30	30
	repose		30	30					
Seasons	spring								30
	summer								
	autumn				0		0		
	winter					0		30	
Literary Form	poetry		30	30				30	30
	prose	0				30		0	
Drama	comedy	30				30			0
	tragedy		30	30			0	20	
Odour	fragrance	30	30	30	30	0	30		30
	unpleasant odour							30	

The amount of agreement between the descriptions of various people is even greater than one might expect.

Table I shows in just what items and to what extent there is agreement for each music number.

An o sign in the table indicates that more than half of the listeners characterized the selection by the term opposite which the o sign stands, not only on one hearing, but on both. 2o indicates that the plurality was in the ratio of 2·1, or more. 3o indicates that the plurality was in the ratio of 3·1, or more. No figure opposite the term indicates that the descriptions recorded in the two hearings did not tally ; in other words, that the two reports were inconsistent. The large number of 3o's is evidence of the fact that most of the hearers agreed in their descriptions of the music, particularly within certain groups. This would mean that there is a definite meaning attached to these terms when used to describe music. It means in addition that the description which is given when hearing the music one time is, in general, the same as the description given when hearing the music at another time.

It would seem that odour and colour do not have this discriminating value. Taste, weight, and the seasons also are not useful as compared with the others. It is a little surprising that weight does not show greater differentiating value, as it is a term one commonly finds in descriptions of music. Colour and the seasons would perhaps show a little more agreement if they were arranged in pairs as the other terms were. For example, spring opposed to autumn, summer opposed to winter, would doubtless show more consistent usage. Likewise the selection of one of several colours does not show the consistency found in other. groups. Those terms which define linear form, distance, temperature, movement, literary form, dramatic form, and odour give more consistent results. In discussing the work at the time, odour was the one group to which the listener greatly objected, saying that they could see no connexion between that and music. However, in the tabulated results it is used very often and with greater consistency than any other set of terms. It seems a little surprising that light and grey do not show more agreement. These terms, like weight, are very commonly used by the music critics.

Some comparisons are more definitely associated with music than others. This fact is brought out by a comparison of the reliability of each type of figure. The reliability is calculated by taking the sum of all the times that observers marked the same simile on second hearing which each marked on first hearing of the selection ; multiply this figure by 2, and divide by the total number of occurrences of that simile in all records. Table II shows the relative reliability of each simile.

TABLE II.—TABLE SHOWING RELIABILITY IN INDIVIDUAL USE OF SIMILES.

Similes.	Per cent Reliability.	Deviation between individuals.	Rank Order.
Temperature . .	83	4	1
Odour . . .	81	26	2
Movement. . .	80	6	3
Poetry–Prose . .	78	5	4
Size	77	4	5
Grey . . .	75	19	6
Light . . .	68	15	7·5
Weight . . .	68	11	7·5
Comedy–Tragedy .	67	10	9
Linear . . .	65	29	10
Distance . . .	61	14	11
Taste . . .	60	31	12
Season . . .	53	17	13
Colour . . .	42	59	14

The column-headed Deviation shows the difference in reliability (in percentage) between the highest and the lowest individual record. Six items show more than seventy-five per cent reliability. All but one (season) show more than fifty per cent. The difference of consistency within any group, that is, the deviation between the highest and the lowest individual, is significant. It is notable that the similes which rank highest all show very low deviation, with the single exception of odour. A small deviation would seem to be further evidence of the reliability of the use of these terms.

The number of listeners is too small to allow a comparison of separate selections. Individuals show but little variation in the average totals of consistent report or description. Using as the common denominator 98, which represents the total possible number of consistent descriptions, the individual totals show only a range of from sixty (60) to seventy (70) per cent, a very small range for individual records. Colour, season, taste, and distance keep the total percentage somewhat smaller than it would be otherwise.

TABLE III.—TABLE SHOWING CONSISTENCY OF COLLECTIVE REPORT

Simile.	Per cent Consistency of Collective Report.	Rank.
Odour	·80	1
Movement.	·79	2
Temperature	·77	3
Size .	·76	4·5
Literary form	·76	4·5
Grey	·72	6·5
Linear	·72	6·5
Light	·67	8·5
Weight	·67	8·5
Dramatic Form	·65	10
Distance .	·60	11·5
Taste	·60	11·5
Season	·52	13
Colour	·40	14

The consistency between the two hearings from the standpoint of agreed report, that is, not individual, but collective judgment, is calculated on the basis of a total of 67, the number of selections heard twice (seven), multiplied by the number of persons who heard each twice. Table III shows the consistencies between the two hearings and the rank of each simile.

Table III, like Table II, shows that movement, temperature, size, literary form, greys, linear comparisons, light, and weight similes appear consistently. Just as in the calculation of individual consistency, so in the calculation of consistency of collective judgment, for each record, colour, season, taste, and distance show low consistency.

The two most important factors to be considered in a study of this kind are, first, the consistency with which the terms are used by different people and by the same people at different times, and second, the discriminating value of the similes used, how well do they distinguish one type of music from another. How much meaning or interpretative value is attached to each?

This descriptive method does seem to discriminate very well between different music types, for example, between such a selection as the Overture Miniature from the Nut Cracker Suite and the Ride of the Valkyries. It is particularly noticeable that the descriptions, in terms of similes, of musical selections which are very similar in objective musical attributes are practically identical, e.g. Volunteers' March and Somewhere in Naples are described in exactly the same terms. These are both rhythmic and their fundamental appeal is physical. The volume, tempo, and instrumentation, too, are very like. On the other hand, the Nut Cracker Suite, and the Ride of the Valkyries are described in almost exactly opposite terms, and their music is of opposite kind.

Meditation—Thais, and On Wings of Song, both melodic violin solos, are described in the same terms, excepting that the Meditation is described as *small*, in addition to its other terms, and the other, On Wings of Song, is described as *warm*. These two figures show a differentiating value which does distinguish the two musical selections. A similar instance is shown by comparison of Humoresque, and On Wings of Song. Both are described by *curved lines, warm, poetry, tragedy,* and *fragrance*, but the Humoresque has in addition *small, light, white, near,* and lacks *sweet* and *repose* which characterize On Wings of Song. These descriptions show most adequately the similarity and contrast between the two types of music.

An interesting and useful classification is given by comparing all those selections which are described by the same terms. For example, those selections which practically all persons describe as poetry are the Meditation—Thais, On Wings of Song, the Nut Cracker Suite, and Humoresque. These are all selections for strings with the exception of a little wood-wind in the Nut Cracker Suite. The only one described as prose was the technically difficult Norwegian Echo Song. The selections which were described as being full of movement, or representing movement, are those with obvious rhythm and dynamic force, the Volunteers' March, the Nut Cracker Suite, and the Ride of the Valkyries. On the other hand, those which were described by *repose* are the Meditation—Thais and On Wings of Song, a very different type of music from the preceding group. The same two are the only ones described as *sweet* (in the taste group). There was unanimous agreement that the Ride of the Valkyries was *cold*. It is perhaps the suggestion of the wind which one gets from the insistent diatonic runs and the constant movement that produces this effect.

Only two selections showed marked (3 : 1) consistency in the *weight* simile for the two hearings. These two selections show a nice contrast and clarity in the use of the terms. One, the Humoresque, is defined as *light*, the other, the Ride of the Valkyries, as *heavy*. One cannot dispute this classification. The latter is also defined in proper consistency, as *dark* and *black*.

In linear description, those defined as *straight* are the Volunteers' March and Somewhere in Naples. These are the selections which have a marked and ever-recurring rhythm, which drives straight on to the end. Those described as *curved* are the Meditation, On Wings of Song, the Nut Cracker Suite, Norwegian Echo Song, and Humoresque. Each of these is characterized by shift in movement (movement in the technical sense) and a freedom of rhythm shifting one way or another, according to the melody.

The three selections defined as *small* are those which have small absolute volume, in other words, which are in common terms played softly. Two of them are violin solos, the third is played by string orchestra (with only a minor introduction of the wood wind). They are the Meditation, Humoresque, and the Nut Cracker Suite. On the other hand, those defined as *large* are those which are actually loud, and which include many instruments—the Volunteers' March, Somewhere in Naples and the Ride of the Valkyries.

CONCLUSIONS

The use of similes in describing the effect of the music to which one listens is justifiable. Certain figures of comparison (including size, linear form, movement, temperature, odour, literary form, grey, light) are used with considerable consistency by different individuals when describing the same selections. Some music shows greater uniformity in this regard than does other music (Table I .

Individual consistency from time to time is also great enough to be significant. This means that the explanation and description which the individual gives to himself of the music, is objective enough that it is defined in the same terms the next time it is heard.

Certain similes prove to be more significant, more valuable in discriminating between music types, than others. For example, odour, although being used with remarkable consistency by various listeners and on different occasions, nevertheless does not have any value in differentiating one selection or one type of selection from another. It means practically nothing to say that most music is like a fragrant odour.

Each of the different forms of sensation are represented on the data chart. These show perhaps more explicitly the extent to which the music experience is translated, or interpreted in terms of other sensations. A few other similes are included which relate to personal experience, but not in the form of direct sensations. It is interesting to note the high consistency and reliability of size, line, and movement—all three of which are elements of the kinæsthetic sense. *Weight*, which is also a kinæsthetic term, shows very low descriptive use. There is, however, sufficient suggestion of the use of kinæsthetic terms here to warrant further study of this particular problem.

That the listener usually converts his enjoyment of music into terms of sensations other than those of audition seem evident. He interprets in terms of old experiences. Does the expression, " We do not understand music, we feel it ", mean this unconscious converting of the musical experience into other personal terms with which we are more familiar ? Or does it mean more specifically that the musical experience has a kinæsthetic parallel ?

A large proportion of our music has its most prominent appeal in arousing bodily movements or a tendency to movement. To some people that is the only appeal which music ever makes. The emotional and ideational effects, however, which make up so small part of the total effect of music could scarcely be accounted for on the kinæsthetic basis, but that kinæsthesis is a part of each emotional experience seems certain.

There is no auditory vocabulary, universally understood, whereby musical experiences can be described. We describe them in terms of the responses which the music arouses and in terms of other experiences which the present one resembles or re-arouses. Those terms which are built up of personal sensory experiences, particularly kinæsthetic, are more adequate and are used with greater uniformity than those which depend on the many individual experiential factors, not primarily sensory. The interpretation of music depends, therefore, on the nature of our own experiences—both personal and derived—and our ability to relate the present stimulus to them.

INDEX OF NAMES

INDEX OF SUBJECTS

INDEX OF CHARTS AND TABLES